The Pocket Learner Special Needs Education

The Ultimate Toolkit for Every Parent

and Caregiver of a Child or Adult

with Special Educational Needs and Disabilities

The Pocket Learner Special Needs Education

The Ultimate Toolkit for Every Parent and Caregiver of a Child or Adult with Special Educational Needs and Disabilities

Andrea Campbell

Pocket Learner Publishing

© Copyright Andrea Campbell 2022 - All rights reserved.

The content contained in this book may not be reproduced, duplicated or transmitted without direct written permission from the author or publisher.

Under no circumstances will any blame or legal responsibility be held against the publisher, or author, for any damages, reparation, or monetary loss due to the information contained within this book; either directly or indirectly. You are responsible for your own choices, actions, and results.

Legal Notice:

This book is copyright protected and is only for personal use. You cannot amend, distribute, sell, use, quote or paraphrase any part, or the content within this book, without the consent of the author or publisher.

Disclaimer Notice:

Please note the information contained in this text is for educational and entertainment purposes only. All effort has been executed to present accurate, up-to-date, and reliable, complete information. No warranties of any kind are declared or implied. Readers acknowledge that the author is not engaging in the rendering of legal, financial, medical, or professional advice. The content within this book has been derived from various sources. Please consult a licensed professional before attempting any techniques outlined in this book.

By reading this document, the reader agrees that under no circumstances is the author responsible for any losses, direct or indirect, which are incurred as a result of the use of the information contained within this document, including, but not limited to, errors, omissions, or inaccuracies.

Inspirational quotes – Andrea Campbell's intellectual property

Pocket Learner Publishing

ISBN: 978-1-914997-01-3 (sc)
ISBN: 978-1-914997-02-0 (hc)

I would like to thank my family —

Richmond and Shari

for their inspiration, understanding

and love.

A Note from the Author

I need your help!

If you enjoy the book and want to support our mission to make a difference, here are ways you can help:

1. **Buy a paper copy** - Thirty percent of the proceeds from sales go to Camptys Foundation – a non-profit which provides support for families caring for children with special needs in developing countries. (See more at camptys.org). You can buy the book on Amazon and at most places where books are sold.

2. **Give a copy** - Find someone who could benefit from the content in this book. This includes stepparents, divorcees and adult children in stepfamilies.

3. **Write a review** – I'd appreciate it very much if you could leave a review on the site where you bought the book. Reviews help my books to rank and become more visible to other readers who may benefit from the content.

Preface

Upon making the decision to have children, the parent-to-be begins to dream about their potential new role in life. You imagine taking your child to sports practices, watching them learn an instrument over the years, and proudly celebrating academic accomplishments in school. For some parents, however, when your eagerly awaited child arrives with special needs, you find yourself in a different place, mourning the loss of the quintessential parenting experience you dreamt of.

Many parents need a period to process and slowly work through the stages of grief. They will likely experience intense feelings of denial, anger, negotiation, and depression. Finally, they ideally arrive at a phase where they accept the child and learn to love them.

Unfortunately, some parents remain in denial for an extended period. This is highly counterproductive. A parent in denial does not advocate for the child—they act as though the child has the capability of their peers and may continue in this vein for years. Some families refuse to obtain a professional assessment for the child because of the perceived stigma of a diagnosis. Ultimately, the one who suffers the most is the child who misses out on the immense benefits of early intervention. The family suddenly realizes that the dynamics must change and makes the necessary adjustments. Some parents experience intense anger; this may lead to relationships falling apart. When parents have mostly settled into a state of acceptance, despite the emotions related to the grief process occasionally resurfacing, they start to dream again. They accept the child and are ready to advocate and fight for what they believe is best for the child. They lavish love on their child and can now appreciate the talents and abilities to which they had previously been blind.

As a parent of a special child, you unwittingly receive a new title: advocate. You learn quickly what it entails as you navigate life with or without your child in tow. The process makes you stronger, but this strength certainly does not nullify worry or self-doubt. The diagnosis of a learning disability does not necessarily signify the end of your world as you know it, but one must now proceed with an exceptionally high learning curve. No two children present the same challenging behaviors or learning difficulties—this is a good reminder that every person is an individual, unique in their own way. You will receive advice and support from many along the way, some helpful and some not, but it will be your job to figure out what is best for your child.

This book, written by a parent for fellow parents and guardians, provides practical advice to help you prepare for and tackle issues you will likely face while parenting a child with special needs. The material will always come back to asking yourself what is best for your child. You will be invited to use the 6-step approach to figure out the best way to help your child to develop confidence and thrive. In addition, it acts as a source of encouragement and support as you persevere through obstacles and hurdles on your journey.

You will face many challenges and interact with professionals across multiple disciplines, but if you have the right mindset and a can-do attitude, no stretch of this journey will remain insurmountable. The earlier you address your child's needs and take action to intervene, the better the outcome will be. While you may harbor conflicting emotions regarding your child's special needs, children of all abilities must know that they are accepted and loved as they are. By wholly accepting your child, special needs included, you put yourself in the best position to help them progress and achieve the abundant life they so deserve.

Table of Contents

Preface vii

Introduction 1
    My story 1
    Parenting special children 2
    The 6-Step Toolkit 7

Chapter 1 - PERCEPTION: The Journey into HOPE Roadmap 9
    Heart 10
    Optimism 14
    Planning 19
    Enlightenment 22
    Key points of chapter 1 28

Chapter 2 - PREPARATION: The Accelerated FAITH Technique 29
    Fearlessness 30
    Action 35
    Investment 39
    Trust 43
    Harmony 47
    Key points of chapter 2 52

Chapter 3 - PARTICIPATION: The GENTLE Approach Solution 53
    Guidance 54
    Enjoyment 58
    Nurturing 63
    Tenacity 68
    Learning 72
    Empowerment 76
    Key points of chapter 3 80

Chapter 4 - PROGRESS: The JOY Generator Blueprint 81
    Jubilation 82
    Opportunity 85
    Yield 89
    Key points of chapter 4 93

Chapter 5 - PATIENCE: The LOVE Game Strategy 95
    Listening 96
    Originality 100
    Vocalization 103
    Encouragement 107

  Key points of chapter 5 113

Chapter 6 - POTENTIAL: The PEACE Promotion Formula.............. 115
  Practice 116
  Evaluation... 119
  Achievement 123
  Creativity.. 127
  Esteem 131
  Key points of chapter 6 137

Chapter 7 - The Pocket Learner 139
  Origins 140
  What it is... 141
  How it works.. 143
  The Pocket Learner – Key Resource in the Toolkit 150
  Key points of chapter 7 152

Conclusion 153

Other Books You'll Love 159

About the Author... 161

Special Needs Glossary... 163

Further Resources and Works Cited 169

Introduction

It was half past six in the afternoon, and I was just about to pull out of the parking lot of our local botanical gardens. For the past three years, at the same time every Friday, my daughter and I have maintained a rhythm of visiting the parks. This was our quality time. We would drive up in our car, have a snack while enjoying music on our favorite station, walk two miles around the park and watch the birds gathered by the lake.

"How is she?" I heard a stranger ask. My eyes met hers as she smiled and waved to my daughter beside me. She'd already assumed that my child was non-verbal or lacked understanding, so she addressed her query to me, speaking about my daughter in her presence. Nevertheless, I responded, and she grinned and said, "I take care of two of them at work, and they are so lovely!" Various aspects of this encounter were inappropriate, but I had learned to pick my battles, so I engaged with her for a few minutes before driving away.

My story

This book has blossomed out of my personal story. My daughter has Down Syndrome and Autism Spectrum Disorder (ASD). She requires additional care and attention, including frequent visits to care professionals, a tailored curriculum, and help with her self-care. Her learning is slow, but her understanding is sharp, and she is a clever, witty child. I realized early on that my life would change drastically as I became her caregiver and advocate. I've battled every step of the way to access resources, various therapy interventions, and care support. I've challenged government and school officials when necessary. We've spent many nights researching her diagnosis and looking into new developments in the field. Although never-ending, it is a fulfilling job—especially when our labor yields fruit and our child takes another step in her growing independence.

When I realized that my daughter was not progressing in her traditional educational institution, a conversation with her teacher helped me to understand that the teacher would not be able to give her the support she needed. I successfully lobbied for her to change schools. My efforts to support her learning did not stop with this, however. I also developed an educational resource that offered the flexibility she needed to progress academically. I call it the Pocket Learner[1] because it entails placing cards into pockets. The Pocket Learner was so helpful that I decided to market it so that other families could reap its benefits. This multi-award-winning educational development system has become very popular. Its development, inspired entirely by my journey with my daughter, is the antecedent of the 6-step Toolkit, which I will discuss later.

PARENTING SPECIAL CHILDREN

I have gathered vast experience in special needs parenting, and my understanding has grown in leaps and bounds. While I refuse to call myself an expert, I feel that my experience is helpful to parents who are on a similar journey and who, like me, sometimes find themselves groping in the dark. One can

---

[1] Please visit https://pocketlearner.net/ for more information

find many experts with theoretical knowledge, but only a parent truly knows how it feels when everyone else is asleep, but your mind and heart are racing because you are up late, yet again, with care duties or researching and preparing for the next doctor's visit. Parenting through challenges that no one else can see, let alone understand, is incredibly lonely. Parents and caregivers of children with special needs often tread unfamiliar waters requiring extreme courage and perseverance. It does not help that our struggles often plague us in a lonely, uncelebrated realm from the public's view. I hope this book will offer some solace and a sense of togetherness. You are not alone.

When a child has special needs, every facet of parenting is magnified. Play dates become complicated projects that need diplomacy, support, patience, and time. Frequent, expensive, challenging trips to the doctor are the norm. Regular shopping trips are often sprinkled with potential pitfalls and disasters. You are almost always fraught with worry. There is so much to worry about, plan for, and anticipate. You quickly learn the uniqueness of your child's 'special' needs. Many parents agree that parenting a child with special needs is isolating, even with the presence and support of extended family.

These children and you, their parents, like every family, have deep needs: love, support, encouragement, and a loving community. That is precisely what I'm extending to you in the pages of this book. You must know that you are not alone in this—people have done this before and excelled. Their children have thrived, and your family can do the same. I am a mother of a child with special needs. I have navigated this journey and discovered some keys to maintaining a balanced, happy, and wholesome family despite the concerns and uncertainties of having a family member with special needs.

I have been involved in the education sector for over 20 years, supporting and empowering families of children with special needs. Upon becoming the parent of a special child, I was able to experience the phenomenon from a different perspective, which has provided fodder for this book. I have prepared this resource to help families navigate the ambiguous path of raising a child with special needs. Only you will understand the deep heartache, fear, and uncertainty of parenting your child. However, once you can recognize and accept the situation, you are well on your way to finding fulfillment in becoming and being the rock upon which your child can lean as they navigate their way in the world.

Throughout this book, for ease of flow, I will use the term "special child" to refer to a child with special needs. I prefer this over the term "special needs child." I do not wish to undermine the fact that every child is special; I aim to emphasize that a child with a disability is first, and foremost, a child—not a disability.

This book introduces the **Special Education Advancement Toolkit**, a six-step process that inspires, educates, and encourages parents to take necessary steps to show up empowered for their kids, enabling them to run their own race and live their best lives. It is an educational model and guide for parents of children struggling in their early years or who have been diagnosed with special educational needs. The toolkit was inspired by my experience as a mother and the principal caregiver of a child diagnosed with Down Syndrome and Autism Spectrum Disorder (ASD). The Pocket Learner, mentioned above, is the central resource in the Toolkit. The Toolkit covers the roles, responsibilities, and activities that families and other relevant parties must implement to achieve success. The framework revolves around the child, the star in the center, endowed with innate abilities and gifts to share with the world.

The Toolkit advocates early, consistent intervention, collaboration, and access to services. This multifaceted strategy yields optimum results for your special child. As a parent, you must find the courage to get started. This is something you may need to do repeatedly when you lose momentum. Sometimes all you need is to connect with other parents of special children. When my daughter was young, I was fortunate enough to have access to a local parents' group that guided me through some of the available government support. They provided a lifeline when I didn't know where to turn. I also embarked on a learning campaign to ascertain all that I could regarding my child's diagnosis. It's been 15 years, and my daughter has blossomed into a confident young woman.

I am pleased to present this Toolkit to you. I hope that you will find the material helpful and that the framework will prompt you to find sources of support. I acknowledge every child's individuality and uniqueness, but I trust you as the parent to adapt the material to your child's situation. Perhaps your child doesn't have a diagnosis, but they find making or maintaining friendships challenging. Maybe they punch walls when they are angry. Maybe they pull their hair out when upset or throw up when nervous. Only you will know which parts of the Toolkit you can adapt to your child.

We know your most challenging parenting moments aren't those you post on social media. The hardest moments are the days you find yourself alone and exhausted, brokenhearted from an insensitive comment, or staring failure in the face despite gargantuan efforts. These are the moments I want you to hold in the front of your mind as you read this book. All parents have moments of hopelessness and uncertainty. I know how deeply painful yours, as a parent of a special child, have been. I have been there.

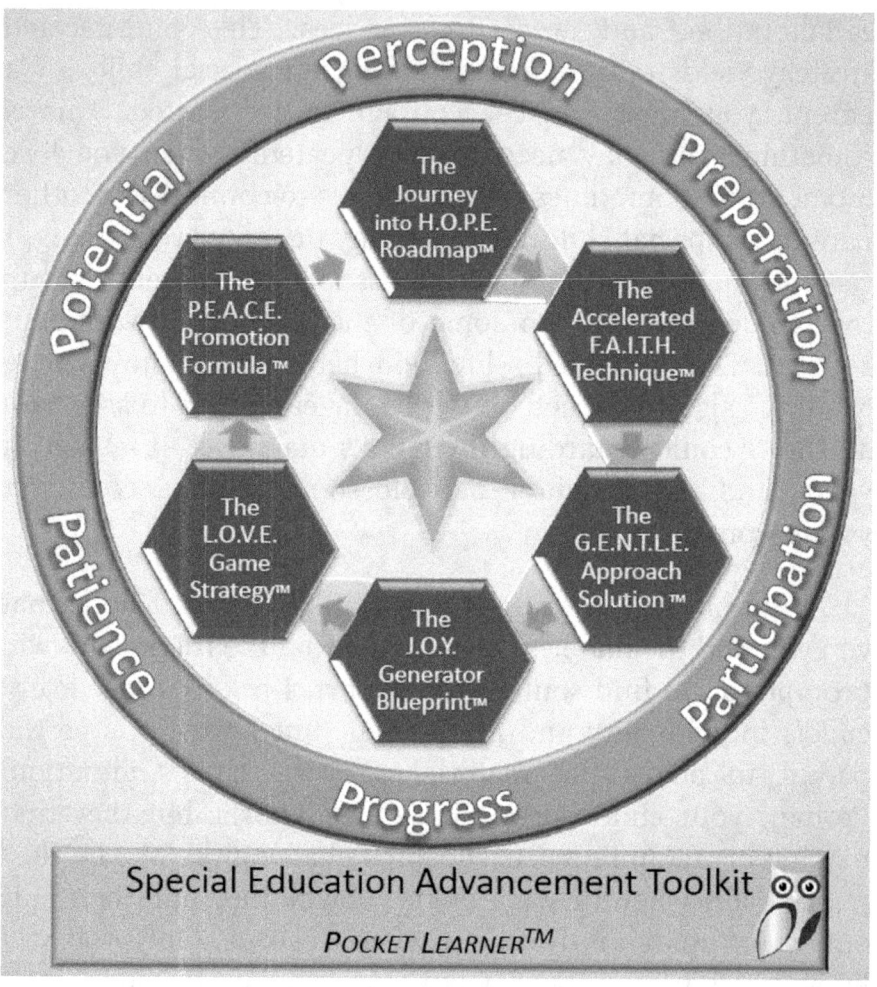

THE 6-STEP TOOLKIT

This book presents a proven systematic method consisting of strategies to help you on your journey. Treat the material as a checklist covering the various factors to consider as you raise your special child. As you progress through the material, you will discover the light at the end of the tunnel for your entire family.

The book introduces six Ps—Perception, Preparation, Participation, Progress, Patience, and Potential—as well as a chapter on the Pocket Learner educational development system. I aim to empower you, as the parent, caregiver, or teacher of a child with special needs and disabilities, by providing valuable information and guidance that will enable you to support your child's learning and development. I hope this book will encourage and guide you as you fulfill your role as a primary or supporting caregiver, or a teacher, of a special child.

Chapter 1

PERCEPTION:
The Journey into HOPE Roadmap

Plan your journey, even if you don't have a ride
—Andrea Campbell

The Journey into HOPE Technique covers early assessments and mindset. The goal of the technique is to attain a position of acceptance, resolve, and hope. The roadmap comprises sections titled **H**eart, **O**ptimism, **P**lanning and **E**nlightenment.

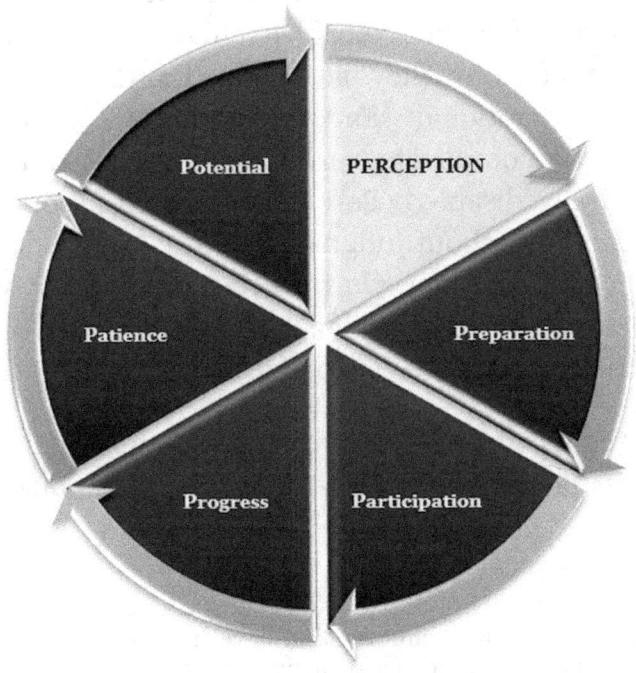

HEART

Being a parent of a special child often entails a lifelong commitment to supporting your child. Once you've grieved the loss of the "normal" child you expected and lovingly embraced the special child you have, you begin a journey of mixed emotions that, while scary at times, often change your life for the better. Love is the glue that holds families together. Statistics show that families caring for a child with special needs are more likely to fall apart.[2] Great parents don't place conditions on love for their children. They lead with love, irrespective of their children's differences or challenges. When a family welcomes a child with special needs, they accept that their physical and emotional support will demand additional time and resources.

It would be amiss of me to say that every parent is immediately accepting and full of love for their disabled child. I have read many accounts of people unwilling or unable to care for their disabled children. I cannot judge those parents for only they have walked in their shoes. It is a profoundly emotional and demanding journey, and undoubtedly a complicated process, to parent children who are profoundly disabled. Parents in this situation have the right to choose without judgment from people who have no experience in the matter. On the other hand, many who, like me, unreservedly love their children and those families might find this toolkit easier to digest.

The responsibility for supporting a child with learning difficulties, physical disability, or sensory impairment is a

---

[2] Sobsey (2004) quotes multiple sources that claim a divorce rate from 70-90% for families with children that have special needs. He compares this to the general average of a 50% divorce rate.

challenging burden. These challenges become even trickier when balancing the needs of other children with those of your special child.

Empowering your special child begins with empowering yourself. You must want to change and be committed to doing all you can for your child and, by extension, your family. A healthy mind is a great place to start. When you work on your mindsets and perceptions, you are better positioned to embark on a journey that benefits your child. You will aim for win-win strategies that foster healthy relationships and genuine partnerships between yourself and professionals. As a caring parent of a special child, you will constantly search for information and services. It is not abnormal to experience feelings of isolation and despair. Sometimes it feels like no one could possibly understand your situation, but this is simply not true.

Unconditional love

Parents of children with special needs continue to free themselves from preconceptions and expectations and learn to love their kids unconditionally. A loving atmosphere is essential for the development of all healthy children; children with special needs are no exception. Children with special needs are more vulnerable and often need help and support their entire lives. Loving your child wholly and deliberately means you embrace them with their disabilities, quirks, and differences. Your love empowers them to overcome challenges, limitations, and obstacles. This increases their confidence and leads to greater cooperation.

Implementing comprehensive therapies and interventions after a child's diagnosis will not suffice if you cannot maintain an atmosphere in which the child feels absolute confidence that they are loved. Focusing on treatment turns the home environment into an unnatural, performative environment. Even if your child is non-verbal, they have strong feelings and may harbor the unspoken belief that something about them needs "fixing," leading to unhappiness and low self-worth. Unfortunately, parents mistakenly believe children with learning difficulties and disabilities do not pick up on as much. Children are aware of when they are treated differently from their peers. They know they "should" be able to do something their peers can and desperately want to perform and be treated like their peers. This situation results in very negative feelings and can damage self-confidence significantly.

The child eventually believes that they are unlovable as they are. As a result, they may internalize the message that they need to act differently to be acceptable, likable, and loved. Indeed, some of these children do not know that they are disabled; they have no perception of it, so they may not pick up on some of what you are saying. However, a child will sense it if they're unloved and find it difficult to achieve happiness. They have a right to be loved and appreciated by their parents for their identities and individuality. Loving, respecting, and accepting your child for who they are, appreciating and valuing each unique aspect of their identity, will give them a feeling of intactness. Your child should feel loved and likable for who they are, unchanged and authentic. This feeling is essential for developing healthy self-esteem and positive self-regard. Moreover, children need to feel that parents appreciate their challenges as a genuine aspect of the child. Parents must communicate respect and appreciation for their child's uniqueness and different ways of learning and doing things.

Love your child wholly and completely. Accept your child as worthy of love, unqualified, and unconditional. Appreciate and acknowledge their value to the world. Don't let them think they need to change somehow to be worthy of love. Love them unconditionally.

The nature of love

It is impossible to love without giving, irrespective of who you are. Love, in essence, is the ability to give without expectation. You need to invest in your relationship with your child. This means spending quality time with them, providing basic material things to satisfy their needs, and, most importantly, providing an atmosphere where the child feels loved and valued. Try to approach parenting from the child's perspective. It does not mean that there will be no rules or that the child runs the show; instead, it means that the child is empowered to be who they are within a safe structure of mutual respect.

Never doubt the child's capacity to understand and follow the rules. Start teaching them early on. My daughter will flaunt the rules whenever she can. Recently, she dropped a napkin on the floor. She knows this behavior is unacceptable, and I didn't have to ask her twice to pick it up. She promptly picked it up and took it straight to the garbage. Of course, the goal is to work toward correcting the child's actions independently without prompting. I would be wrong to pick up the item when she can do it herself. Even if your child is in a wheelchair, you must still teach them not to litter. If your child is non-verbal, you must still use appropriate communication to teach them. The best way is to model good behavior; when that fails, find a quiet time and space to discuss the matter using methods of communication appropriate for your child.

Give them the kind of love you expect them to give you. Teach them to love and remind them that they deserve to be treated lovingly by those around them. Listen and try to understand what is valuable to them. Look for opportunities to learn from other children and adults with special needs respecting them as valued, whole, worthy of love, and deserving of inclusion.

Embrace your child's uniqueness. Make your actions match your words. Don't just tell them; show them that you love them. Love and embrace your child as they are, not for who you'd like them to be.

Think about these questions. Write down detailed answers to them when you are ready:

1) Do you love your special child unconditionally? What would or does this look like?

2) Are you at peace with your child's diagnosis?

3) Do you enjoy the child's company?

4) How do you feel about the sacrifice you make to care for your child? What can you do to come to terms with them? Are there any that you could reconsider at this point in your child's development?

OPTIMISM

Cultivating optimism is essential in parenting children with special needs. Without optimism, it is easy to feel hopeless and helpless about your child's future. Though you might not get everything right all the time, and you feel like you have to put in a ridiculous amount of work to get the slightest improvement, and you might feel like no one in your support community understands how much work you are putting in, your efforts are not futile. Maintaining optimism despite challenges is easier for some parents than for others. This is something that can and must be learned, though. A parent's ability to bounce back from failed attempts and stay optimistic, even if they need a brief period of mourning the failure or changing their approach, will give their child the best chance to aspire and achieve.

The need for optimism

As the parent of a child with special needs, do you feel genuine optimism about their future? Unfortunately, for many parents, hope is rarely inspired by our surrounding environment. The number of children born with special needs is increasing; however, social norms, the school environment, and the medical community seem unfit, ill-equipped, or possibly unwilling to rise to the challenges and realities of special needs. Struggling economies put special needs even further down the list of societal priorities to be addressed. This leaves many parents wrestling with questions: What about our children? What will become of them? What things should they look forward to in the future? Can we dare to hope?

Hope is something we must seek intentionally and diligently. We cannot wait around blaming others who have not given it to us. You do not have this luxury. Your child needs you. Every individual must find a source of hope. There is, however, a reason to hope—your child offers a unique contribution to the world. Your job is to find and nurture it.

Discover your child's talent. Why does the world *need* your child? With perseverance, passion, and patience on your part, you will almost certainly be blown away by how much your child can accomplish. When you nurture their talent, you also nurture their social skills, feelings of well-being, and confidence. It is your job to show your child and the world what your child can contribute to the world. I cannot overstate the value of supporting and helping our special children find activities that tap into their talents, strengths, and passions. The late South-African Archbishop Desmond Tutu summarized this well when he said, "Hope is being able to see that there is light despite all the darkness."

Expect success and have a positive outlook. Remember that your child can thrive just like everyone else if you nurture their talents and passions. Think about and write down answers to these questions:

1) How are you keeping hope alive?

2) How are you encouraging your child to find their passion and purpose?

3) Why does the world need your child?

4) Do you genuinely believe you can succeed in your endeavor to help this child become the best version of themselves?

5) If the answer to the previous answer is yes, what are you doing to demonstrate your belief in your child's ability to thrive and grow?

Jamal Robinson—A case for optimism

For over fifteen years, I have been involved in several parent groups and interacted with multiple agencies focusing on children with special needs. In that period, I have met people from all walks of life and heard many optimistic stories from parents of children with special needs. One particular story has stayed with me. At the age of two years, Jamal was diagnosed with autism. Fifteen years later, his parents feel more optimistic about his future, despite all the unknowns and challenges.

Jamal's immune system was compromised, and he was constantly sick. He was non-verbal and couldn't communicate even the most basic needs to his parents. He cried continuously and screamed for hours, hoping to be understood. One terrifying day Jamal, approximately 15 years old, ran away from home. After resolving this crisis, Jamal's parents resorted to round-the-clock supervision. Faced with unsustainable solutions to immense challenges, how could this family find hope and optimism? A paintbrush came to their rescue.

Jamal couldn't hold a fork properly at the time, but he grabbed a paintbrush from his mother and slowly started dabbing paint onto a canvas one day. Curious and happy that he had taken an interest in something other than his iPad and videos, his parents searched for an art teacher.

Jamal started slowly, painting for one minute only. He was, however, proud of his paintings and often stood next to the canvas for a photo. Jamal struggled to follow formal instructions but was open and willing to learn, working in small increments. The teacher built on each gain and reinforced it. Jamal was noticeably frustrated when his pictures failed to take form, but everyone was happy to see that he had taken an interest in a craft. He sometimes threw away the brush, but ultimately he persisted, and his perseverance paid off.

When Jamal had produced 100 paintings, his parents decided to hold a fundraiser to pay for his therapy and make space. In addition to the paintings, they printed 1,500 greeting cards from the images. The event was successful with the selling of 48 pictures and all the cards. Jamal received many compliments from people who supported the fundraiser, and he was visibly overwhelmed even though he may not have fully understood the day's events. Imagine what it did to his self-esteem to have people validate his talents and buy his paintings!

The fundraiser deepened Jamal's sense of accomplishment, passion, and pride. Jamal's confidence grew in leaps and bounds over the years, and whenever his art was displayed, appreciated, or sold, he felt a tremendous sense of accomplishment.

Jamal is now twenty years of age, but he is only nine developmentally. He still has many challenges and may never become completely independent. He is not very expressive verbally, but the look on his face when he sees one of his paintings hanging in a local business around the neighborhood is priceless. This was the spark of optimism his family needed to keep going.

Jamal's experience shows that there is always a reason and a season for hope; things will get better if we keep hope alive. Your child has a hidden passion, talent, or interest. Maybe they can swim, paint, dance or play an instrument. Spotting their skills might take time, but keep looking! Every day is a new opportunity to support and encourage your child lovingly.

PLANNING

Every family needs to plan, but planning is crucial for families of children with special needs. These plans require special thought and dedication because they often involve finding just the right professionals and can involve great expense. Many parents struggle to discern where to start. The answer is determined by your child's age and diagnosis as well as your financial and family situation.

The following is an essential guide that can help you. This list isn't comprehensive, but it is a checklist focusing on the core issues parents should address. When necessary, ask for help. Ask family, friends, educational personnel, and health professionals working with the child.

Therapy and care

You are the primary caregiver for your child. You play a huge role in their lives, but you'll need direction and support from professionals at some point. The following thoughts and questions about care and therapy will guide you toward the best answers and decisions:

1) Which healthcare professionals is your child already seeing? Do you understand what they are saying about your child? Have you asked them questions that you may have about your role in interventions? Which professionals would you like your child to continue with? If with all of them, that's great. If, however, some of them cause hesitation, consider finding another practitioner to fill that role.

2) Which therapeutic interventions is your child receiving? Are these sufficient, effective, and worth

your financial resources? If not, should you consider others that better address your child's needs?

3) Which medications is your child taking? Which ones should you stop, and which ones should you continue?

4) What are your child's scheduled activities? Are they adding value to your family?

5) Who are the family members and friends interacting with your child? Are they supportive? Do they have a basic understanding of your child's diagnosis? Is it necessary to share information with them?

Educating yourself on government-provided financial supports such as Medicaid and Social Security is also essential. You don't need to become an expert, but if you don't acquire a basic understanding of these programs, you may miss out on opportunities that could benefit you and your family. At the very least, you should study their core benefits and ascertain whether your child qualifies to access them. It is crucial to start the process early as some support systems may offer wider coverage before your child reaches age eighteen.

Vocational training

Start by talking to the school guidance counselor if your child is a teenager who attends secondary school. If your child goes to a special education school, the counselor is most likely familiar with academic and vocational opportunities in your area. You can also contact organizations online by typing in your child's diagnosis and adding the word 'support'. Some of these organizations may not provide training opportunities but may have a database that could be helpful to you in finding resources and outlets. Local community colleges are an excellent resource too. Many have classes—specially designed for students with special needs. These institutes may offer additional opportunities for your child to excel.

Employment

This step may not be an option for all parents or children, but if your child can work, help them find employment. You may be able to start an online or offline business venture with your child. You can create a foolproof plan that ensures your child has a progression path. Some parents can create businesses to benefit other children with special needs along with their children. Such companies may focus on hiring young adults with special needs. Several existing businesses in our communities employ young people and older adults with special needs and disabilities. Think, for example, of Goodwill Industries, which operates here in the United States.

Legal and financial planning

A legal plan allows you to protect, transfer and control your assets during your lifetime and after you are gone so that your child can access the resources they need to live a fulfilling life. Your legal plan also ensures the implementation of any comprehensive special-needs programme, even if you can no longer make decisions for your child.

There are two critical decisions to be made when a child with special needs reaches the age of eighteen: Medical decisions and financial decisions. First, you'll have to decide whether guardianship is appropriate for your family or if there's a more desirable alternative. At eighteen, your child becomes eligible for Social Security based on their financial security now and in the future. If you plan to support and care for your child long-term, you should consider making a Social Needs Trust where you can save money (including financial gifts received) for your child. Most are complicated, and only an attorney familiar with these issues should draft them.

Future guardians - This is a question that every parent grapples with, especially in times of medical uncertainty for the parent or guardian. Whom do you trust to take over if you can no longer care for your child? Simply finding and choosing a capable individual is not the end of the task either. Once you have found a competent individual, you must educate them and let them know what it takes to be a guardian of a child with special needs. The conversation should be open and honest to allow the potential guardian to consider the responsibilities before committing.

ENLIGHTENMENT

You may need some time to adjust following your child's diagnosis, and that's okay. Everyone reacts differently to such news, and there is no right or wrong way to feel. Of course, you will have many positive and negative emotions, but please remember that acquiring a diagnosis is tremendously positive. It is a colossal first step in addressing your child's needs. Once you've received the diagnosis and allowed yourself to process and deal with the emotions, you're ready to move forward in researching and discerning an action plan.

A medical provider or the school district may diagnose children with a disability. However, being diagnosed with a disability does not guarantee services under the Individuals with Disabilities Education Act (IDEA)[3]. According to SpecialEducationGuide.com—an online resource for parents and educators in the special education arena—the evaluation team must also determine if the disability impacts the child's educational progress and qualifies the child for specially designed instruction.

Conduct research and educate yourself

Learn as much as you can about the diagnosis. The more you know, the better you will be able to cope and manage for the long haul. Here are some questions you can focus on:

- How does the diagnosis manifest itself?

- What behavioral challenges, if any, should you anticipate?

- How can you help your child cope with or manage their condition?

- What learning challenges should you expect?

- What rights does your child have when they attend school? What accommodations does your child need? Is the school able and willing to provide them? Does your child have any legal protection in qualifying for the necessary accommodations?

- Do you have the time and energy to advocate for necessary accommodations that your child is not legally granted? Can you get professional help in advocating for this?

---

[3] Please visit https://sites.ed.gov/idea/ for more details on United States education accommodations of children with special needs.

People say information is power. However, you'll be powerless if you do nothing with that information. The correct information will help you understand the details of your child's diagnosis, any additional issues they may have, and actions you must take on a medium or long-term basis to ensure they maintain good health. Every child is unique, so don't expect your child to behave like other children with a similar diagnosis. Learning about the specifics of the diagnosis is necessary because some information might apply to other children and not your child. While researching, please remember that experts did not write all the information you find online. Be selective with your sources and cross-check as much as possible. It's important to ensure that your child is learning; for this to happen, you need to understand the dynamics of special education.

To find specific information that relates to your child's condition, here are some suggestions:

- Join a local support group or parent's group.

- Talk to other parents and guardians of children with the same condition. Ask them what they've found useful and the details about what works for them.

- Ask your physician, therapists, and other professionals for recommended literature.

- Seek out organizations and charities relevant to your child's diagnosis.

- Join parent groups online and engage with members.

Connect with other parents

You'll need to find your tribe and stay close to people who understand. Their relevant experience may or may not be helpful but will most certainly motivate you to keep trying. Read their stories and listen when they speak. Developing camaraderie based on your shared experiences will significantly strengthen you when you feel alone. Join a local support group or parent's group when you feel ready. You may receive tremendous encouragement and often practical help by talking to another parent whose child has a similar condition.

When you engage with others, you will feel less lonely on your journey as a parent of a child with special needs. My daughter attends a school for children with disabilities. It is beautiful when parents gather at the school gates to compare notes. It feels like we have found long-lost speakers of our unique language. We celebrate small victories that typical parents would overlook or take for granted. We talk about things others may find disgusting, such as how often our children go to the toilet and the consistency of their bowel movements—matters others may find repulsive, yet they are integral to our daily lives. That is the power of community and sharing struggle. Most parents admit the tremendous help they receive when talking to another parent whose child has a similar condition.

You may also benefit from the following resources: researching services provided by local authorities, reading relevant blogs, joining parent forums, watching relevant videos online, visiting online communities, and creating a support group. If you need an outlet, you can talk to a counselor, call a helpline, talk to someone who understands—a partner, family member, or friend, write a blog, and create videos to share your journey with others.

Speak to educational and health professionals

Become familiar with the 504 plan system. This program is designed to ensure that all children with special needs in the United States public elementary and secondary school systems receive the necessary accommodations to access the learning environment and achieve academic success. Alongside the 504 plan is the Individualized Educational Plan (IEP)—a program for children who need specialized instruction. The plan requires specific measurements of growth and is more demanding on a school. Please note that these documents do not legally bind private schools in the United States, but they are often willing to set up a similar framework. You must discern whether you trust the school to act in your child's best interest as it will be you, rather than the state, requesting accommodation that demands the school's time and resources. Be sure to write everything down to prepare for unanticipated school personnel changes.

Your efforts may not make a difference to everyone, but that's not your goal. Your goal is to do what will most increase the chances of your child's success. Write down questions with possible suggestions you can discuss with parents and professionals. Keeping a journal or a running list of questions is also essential. Keep notes and relevant articles. You may want to share this information with the professionals who work with your child. Notes and relevant reports will give them a head start.

Ask for written information. Written information from doctors and professionals will go a long way. Also, be sure to let the professionals know upfront that you want as much information and resources as they may be able to offer. Most professionals avoid overwhelming parents of children with special needs. They will wait until you let them know you are ready for in-depth information or details about a particular subject.

Avoid people who make definitive statements. Be cautious about taking advice from people who have opinions about your child's skills and abilities, especially when those are negative or limiting. No one can predict the future. Besides, many factors determine what a child will become and their accomplishments later in life.

Always ask if someone else can help. If the person you are currently working with is unavailable, you'll need help from someone else. It's good to ask doctors and professionals for other trustworthy names in the field. As you enlighten yourself, you must focus on the following questions:

- How will your child's diagnosis impact their education, movement, development, memory, and behavior?

- What interventions and services should you prioritize for this diagnosis?

- Which professionals or therapists are most knowledgeable about your child's diagnosis?

Understanding the basics and filtering through the information will help you find answers to build a profile for your child. The profile can list their symptoms, medical conditions, necessary therapy plans, required health professionals, and educational needs.

KEY POINTS OF CHAPTER 1

> Put your HEART into the process; start by cultivating an environment of love for your child—be deliberate about this. Choose OPTIMISM and find hope in your child's talents, abilities, and passions. Determine why the world needs your child and help your child live fully. Be intentional. PLAN for your child's success in school, extracurricular activities, and therapy opportunities. ENLIGHTEN yourself by learning as much as possible about your child's diagnosis and the plethora of available resources locally and online. You are well into your Journey into HOPE.

Chapter 2

PREPARATION:
The Accelerated FAITH Technique

The journey of a thousand miles begins in the mind
—Andrea Campbell

The Accelerated FAITH Technique highlights the attitudes and initial actions required for the successful implementation of the program. This section will explore **F**earlessness, **A**ction, **I**nvestment, **T**rust, and **H**armony.

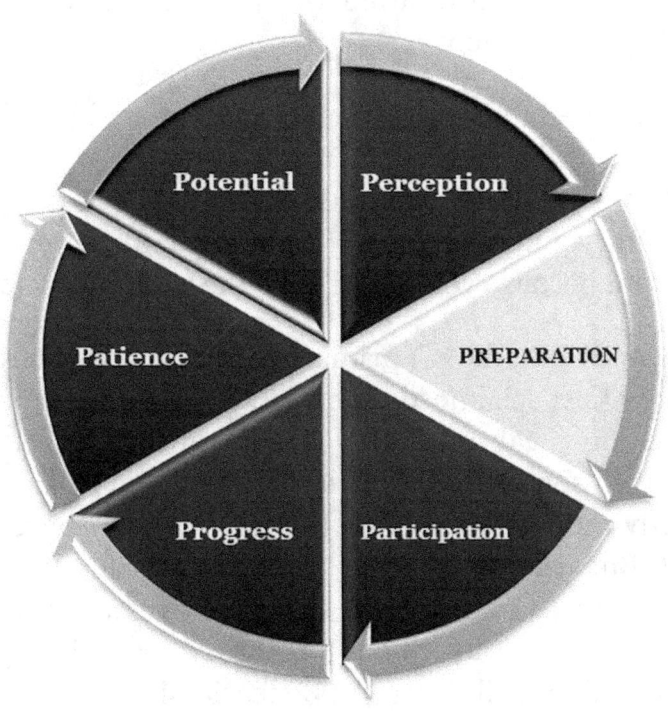

FEARLESSNESS

As parents and primary caregivers, we understand our children best. We know when they are unwell or just tired. As parents of special children, we are in tune with their moods, needs, and wants. We know if they would benefit from an electronic device or a trampoline. School and health professionals see the children for a few hours and have a limited understanding of how the diagnosis affects the child.

When the parents' views differ from those of teachers and health professionals, life becomes stressful, and progress may reach a temporary stand-still. Many parents will agree that they've gone through their fair share of struggles with health professionals, educators, and the government system. Parents of children with special needs constantly battle anxiety while juggling appointments and interventions for therapy and medical treatments, running a household, and sustaining employment.

As the parent of a special child, you are on high alert and may find it difficult to relax. You may constantly be on the lookout for the unexpected—watching for triggers or positioning yourself to take a quick exit from yet another social event because your child is on the verge of an episode.

Finances can be a primary concern too. Parents of children with special needs generally have higher expenses in insurance, medical costs, travel, and subsistence. Raising a special child sometimes feels like running a marathon with a constantly moving finish line because you can never get to the end. But we do it anyway, and we do it fearlessly. As a committed and loving parent, you must fight for resources and support for your child. You are your child's greatest advocate. Pull out all the stops. Be fearless!

Fight for their education

Children with special needs have the right to obtain supplemental services or accommodations in the public education system. According to federal legislation, every child has the right to an appropriate education in the best possible setting. Some laws were written to support children with special needs in public schools. They include:

- IDEA – Individuals with Disabilities Education Act (1975)
- Rehabilitation Act (1973) – Section 504
- ADA – Americans with Disabilities Act (1990)

The eligibility criteria are different in every state. The procedures and available services also differ from state to state. Studying these laws and how they apply in your state is essential to find the best route to advocate for your child's education.

Fight for therapy

Always request an assessment of your child before determining the necessary intervention. The assessment will rely on input from your child's school, an educational psychologist, a doctor, social services, and your family and caregivers. The assessment is a detailed document covering a range of skills, including speech and language, learning, psychological testing, and behavioral analysis. You may have the option of an assessment covering various domains, or you may need to arrange multiple assessments from independent professionals. Both of these options will require time and money. Know your insurer's policies—you can sometimes obtain financing even if your insurer's network does not include the specialist your child needs. Ask other families in forums who use the same insurance. If you have limited coverage, it never hurts to ask professionals if they can offer any financial aid.

When you begin therapy, keep updated and written evaluations in a safe place. The evaluation reports should include observations by doctors, teachers, family members, and caregivers. With the results from these evaluations, you'll be able to demand a range of support, including physical therapy, speech, and language therapy, occupational therapy, behavioral therapy, or the allocation of a classroom aid.

The evaluation results give you the right to an Individualized Education Plan for your child (IEP). You have the right to participate in the creation of your child's IEP. You also have the right to dispute and appeal the findings and conclusions of the assessment. If your child attends a public school, the school administrators must give you the necessary information to appeal.

Depending on your child's needs and evaluation findings, you may be referred to a speech therapist, occupational therapist, or neurodevelopmental pediatrician. This often requires numerous phone calls, office visits, and letters from various professionals before settling on the right one.

Fight for recognition

The state or the school system may ignore some rare conditions. Official recognition, however, gives a child access to opportunities and accommodations to help them grow and develop closely in line with their class. A child may be able to perform some tasks within a typical classroom environment, for example, reading a sentence during a group activity, after having had a one-on-one pull-out session with a classroom aid or key worker.

Some special needs are not obvious. Some children can walk, run and jump without any outward display of their disability. They appear neurotypical to the untrained eye. However, these children may also need extra support and present as much of a challenge as visibly disabled children. I recently witnessed a friend's pain when her 13-year-old autistic son ran away during a park visit. After five horrifying hours of searching for the boy, she learned someone had spotted him on a train track and called the police. The search took several hours partly because of the public's inability to recognize his disability. Needless to say, this episode could have ended very differently.

Hidden disabilities also make accessing services even more difficult. I was recently in line with my family at the airport. We didn't have to wait long because Down Syndrome is a visible disability. However, a family with a boy on the autism spectrum (ASD) did not receive such treatment. It seemed, to the untrained eye of the officer, that their child was simply disruptive, but with my experience, I could tell that there was more to the picture.

If you are concerned that your child's hidden disability may cause a similar encounter, bring a letter from your doctor. Also, many airport personnel in Europe and North America receive training to recognize non-visible disabilities. Before travel, you can obtain the Sunflower Lanyard by mail globally free of charge from Heathrow Airport in the United Kingdom. Your child can wear it, or you can find another way to display it as you travel. It allows airport personnel to accommodate individuals with hidden disabilities better. Before your trip, you may wish to research similar accommodations in the region within which you will travel.

Fight for access

Your child deserves to feel loved and welcomed in school, places of worship, commercial centers, and social venues. When my daughter was four, we attended a weekly church service. I stopped when I realized they were isolating her from the other children during Sunday school. I spoke to the Sunday-school teacher, but the behavior continued, so I took my child and left. It surprised me that people who profess a faith of love and care were so out of touch and unkind to vulnerable children.

Like everyone else, our children deserve to play at the park and visit zoos, museums, and movie theaters. Do you want a movie theater to play a sensory-friendly movie once in a while? Ask them! It's okay to ask for improved accessibility to parks for differently-abled children. Improved access means greater inclusion. Your special child is a member of society and has every right to participate in all the available amenities.

When you fight for access, you create opportunities for your child to learn, grow, and interact with the world outside their home. This, in turn, benefits all of society. It is not always easy to achieve what we want for ourselves and our children. As contemporary society grows more insular and profit-driven, we must battle for services, recognition, and access. I wish I could say it gets easier with time, but unfortunately, the battle with educational, health and government systems will continue. Resources are limited, so you must be creative and strategic. Pick your battles; our children are definitely worth the fight.

ACTION

When you take action to help a child with special needs, you invest in their future. You empower them to be independent. Your goal as a parent is to ensure your child has the appropriate tools. Don't be surprised when they begin to overcome seemingly impossible obstacles and become stronger and more resilient.

Your approach and response to challenges impact your child directly. Approach problems armed with a positive attitude and a go-getter spirit, and you will inspire your child to aim higher even if some obstacles remain a challenge. Below are some good practices as we prepare to take action to empower your special child.

Be proactive - A proactive person pre-empts issues, makes decisions, and takes action to resolve problems or achieve goals. It means you will need to face uncomfortable situations and make reasonable requests for your special child to receive fair treatment. For example, you may need to ask the school to ensure that your child sits at or near the front of the class if the child has issues with vision or hearing. Even when your child has an Individual Education Plan, these matters can be overlooked if they are not specifically raised. You must be willing to stand behind your requests.

It is also necessary to be proactive in social settings. I recall my daughter and I attended an event where she sat beside an elderly lady. The host brought a cup of tea for the woman, and she kindly accepted it. I instantly switched places with my daughter because I could see an accident waiting to happen. This is a prime example of how parents of special kids must be alert to spot potential trouble. The incident occurred at a social event but could easily have happened in an educational, healthcare, or another type of institution. Parents must be proactive in anticipating hazards and take steps to avoid them.

Set goals - The ability to set realistic and achievable goals is a crucial life skill for success. Write down everything you want to accomplish when you attend meetings. Set your priorities and be clear about what you are willing to negotiate. Recognize the need to be flexible to adjust and adapt your goals according to changing circumstances and restrictions. When you adopt a relaxed attitude, you are better positioned to handle emerging challenges you will undoubtedly encounter on your unique journey.

Ask for help - Families of disabled children, young people, and adults benefit greatly from solid support systems. Don't be afraid to seek help; reach out to others for support when you need it. Demonstrate to your child how to ask for help in familiar settings and help them develop and nurture good relationships. Share examples of people needing help, how they got it, and why it was good to ask for help. Present your child with role-play scenarios that might require assistance. Always remember to show gratitude to those who help you and acknowledge that they share out of their own limited time and resources.

Communicate regularly with teachers - We live in an era of consistent budget cuts and inadequate school funding. More than ever, your role in your child's education is crucial. Sitting back and watching from the sidelines as someone else takes responsibility for your child's educational welfare is not a viable option. You can and must play an active role alongside your child's teachers to ensure that your child receives all the support services they need and for which they are eligible.

Advocating for your child's needs can be overwhelming. Superior negotiation skills and constant communication are necessary to defend your child's need for an excellent education. When communicating, be clear about your goals and actively listen. Avoid confrontation and, instead of complaining, try to be solution-oriented. School officials may have differing opinions about the best educational provision for your child. You might have a different perspective or fresh ideas on problem-solving. Share your thoughts gently but be assertive where required. Be a good listener, ask for clarification where necessary, and take notes. Irrespective of any distractions, you must endeavor to stay focused. Educators are dealing with multiple children with different needs- acknowledge their limitations, but remember you are only responsible for one child—your child.

For this reason, the meeting should be about your child. Say their name frequently and avoid drifting into generalizations. You must also avoid the urge to fight complicated battles. Instead, focus on what needs to be done today and forge a way toward a solution together.

Find appropriate ways to thank educators. Bringing a plate of fresh-baked brownies to a meeting is a great way to quickly communicate that you recognize your child's teacher is likely working overtime and show your appreciation.

Persevere - Perseverance allows you to keep going despite challenges and failures and affords you the flexibility to change course if things aren't working. When frustration sets in, communicate to the respective body in writing. If they fail to respond, try again. Navigating the system can be exhausting, but you must not give up on something that could impact your child's future.

Engage with professionals - The ideal relationship between parents of children with special needs and professionals working in the field has the characteristics of honesty, trust, and mutual respect. You and the professional can share ideas and information about the most appropriate care, relevant educational programs, and medical interventions. If a professional's vocabulary is overly technical, ask for clarification and write down the answers. Likewise, taking notes is imperative when therapy or medication is being discussed or prescribed.

Both parties must be transparent and forthright about critical concerns. Recognize that you both have valuable information and skill to contribute to the relationship. For example, you thoroughly understand your child's unique routine, needs, strengths, development, progress, history, condition, and behaviors. On the other hand, the professional contributes specialist information and expertise related to their discipline. The professional also offers the context of a long practice of working with children similar to your own and seeing them grow and succeed. Work together to use all of this for the benefit of your child.

It is good to reach out to other parents as you seek to identify a specialist for your child. They may know surgeons, dentists, and therapists who have worked successfully with their children. Before meeting with teachers, professionals, and other parents, write down your questions and concerns. Look for knowledgeable specialists about your child's diagnosis, willing to collaborate with other doctors, and with

Preparation: The Accelerated FAITH Technique

whom you feel secure and at ease. Finally, consider the advice you receive for therapy, interventions, and treatment programs and measure it against your commitments, schedules, and financial capacity. Sometimes it's impossible to follow up on all the available advice; you must use discernment, keeping the bigger picture in mind.

INVESTMENT

As parents of children with special needs, we want good outcomes for our children. This objective requires us to go beyond the basics and secure additional resources—tangible and intangible—to help our children learn academically and develop life skills. Investing in appropriate intervention and materials for our children based on their abilities and interests is good practice. Investment isn't just about your child's current situation; it's about preparing them for the future. We seek appropriate tools to help our children learn, thrive, and be happy.

Parents must invest carefully and choose the best intervention for their child's unique needs. According to the Learning Disability Association of America, "nonverbal learning disabilities are associated with impairment in motor skills, visual-spatial organizational memory, and social abilities." There is a broad spectrum of characteristics that non-verbal learners may have in those three areas. There is, therefore, no ideal mix of resources or support for all children. As a parent, you will know what is best for your child and do what you can to feasibly secure the necessary materials and services. Depending on where you live, you may be able to access some therapy and resources free of cost or at a subsidized rate. In addition, some agencies work with the government to provide affordable or accessible buy-in therapy for children with special needs.

In some cases, medical insurance will cover a portion of buy-in-therapy. However, many of us are not so lucky and will need to invest in products and services for our children. Sometimes we may have to resort to online options if we need special services unavailable in our local vicinity. Research the best possible choice for your child, and don't be afraid to travel or think outside the box if you cannot find a local professional with proven success. You risk needlessly spending money and energy, and you could also miss out on the opportunity to shape your child's critical developmental years by wasting time with subpar professionals simply because they were cheaper or more easily accessible.

Therapy

Here's a list of buy-in therapy in which you can invest:

Occupational therapy - An occupational therapist will help your child with day-to-day life skills, including dressing, oral, motor, and sensory processing, handwriting, feeding, play, and social interaction. In addition, an occupational therapist evaluates delays or difficulties and helps your child successfully use various body parts, including arms, wrists, and legs, thus developing agility, coordination, and core strengths.

Art therapy - This therapy combines art and psychological therapy to help children deal with emotional or mental problems, anxiety or depression, addictions, loss, trauma, social challenges, and family issues. An art therapist helps children find meaning through illustrations using their unique approaches and imagination. A child may not express themselves verbally, but art therapy gives them an outlet to express thoughts and feelings.

Visual therapy - If your child's vision needs improvement, you'll need the services of visual therapists. Visual therapy focuses on perceptual-cognitive weaknesses and visual-motor skills. It treats learning-related visual challenges, lazy eyes, double and computer vision, and other visual problems. Many children with special needs have benefited from the help of vision therapy-certified optometrists. Vision therapists help children focus and read better through computer equipment and optical devices.

Listening therapy - Listening therapy is also known as auditory training, stimulation or integration training. By listening to guided music, children can improve their listening skills. Listening therapy also assists with social behavior, communication skills, language, and creativity. It also improves concentration, attention, and focus.

Neurofeedback – This exercises the brain. It trains a child in self-regulation. Special sensors are attached to a child's scalp to record brain waves over a certain period. The process is non-invasive and painless because no voltage is used. The hair also remains intact. The child watches a video game that reveals brain waves. Neuropathy helps with sleep difficulties, bed wetting issues, nightmares, anxiety, depression, headaches and migraines, attention, and focus.

Psychotherapy - Psychotherapy can be a life-changing experience that can help improve your child's mental health, overcome social or emotional challenges, and fulfill their potential. Most children with learning disabilities have intellectual impairment ranging from mild to moderate; psychotherapy can often help.

Private tutors - The public school system is ill-equipped to assist with the vast spectrum of challenges children with special needs face. As a parent, you should consider filling the gaps in education if you can afford it. Without a trained teacher, do your best at home and secure help from family and friends. Many children with learning disabilities get overwhelmed in group-learning settings and may fail to thrive academically despite having the ability. A well-designed private tuition program identifies a child's learning style, builds their confidence, and tailors a program suited to the child for parents to follow. It is delivered in an environment conducive to learning and void of triggers.

Programs available in-store and online -The internet contains various programmes designed to teach children with special needs. Among them is the SCERTS® Model—a research-based educational approach and multidisciplinary framework to support children and persons with Autism Spectrum Disorder (ASD) and related disabilities and their families. The model builds competence in Social Communication, Emotional Regulation, and Transactional Support.

The following chapter will introduce the Pocket Learner System I developed to help my daughter build her vocabulary and learn to read. The system now includes numeracy, and it is enabling families across the globe to boost their children's learning. Suffice it to say that the system is revolutionary and widely used in different countries.

Equipment - Other resources that may require investment include specialist bikes and trikes, trampolines, ipads or tablets, computer games, adapted utensils, and toys. Some children may benefit from a weighted blanket to help them sleep. Others need special footwear or clothing. When you have a differently-abled child, you can expect to spend more even if you do not purchase specialist equipment. For example, you may need an adapted vehicle or budget for taxis rather than using public transport to attend therapy or extra-curricular activities.

The effect of a reasonable investment in your child will have a lasting impact on their future. So do not hesitate to invest time and resources in your child.

TRUST

I have heard parents say they did not trust themselves to look after their children. This sentiment applies to parents of neurotypical children and those of special children. Having a young child to care for, especially without a support network, can be scary. It is even more daunting when that child has special needs. Parenting, for the most part, is not taught in institutions; it is life that teaches us, and many of us did not learn how to parent a special child from our own families. Once we adapt to the novelty and demands of the role, most parents do a fine job by trusting their intuition and accessing available support. It is indeed true that it takes a village to raise a child. In this section, I'd like to encourage you to trust your ability to raise your child and advocate on their behalf.

Your mindset

The beliefs we have about our abilities and potential build our mindset. Our mindset controls our behavior and the level of success we achieve. But it's also true that everyone can work on their mindset, improve it, and transform their thinking with the right strategies. As a parent with a child who needs additional care, you cannot afford to have a rigid mindset. The right mindset recognizes that you can control your thinking patterns. You can manage your actions and make decisions that result in positive outcomes. As you build self-belief, your positive mindset rubs off on your child and other family members. The right attitude benefits your relationship with your child as you become a flexible, positive thinker.

As you explore and learn how powerful your mind is, you open yourself to endless possibilities. You may have heard the saying, 'the only prison that exists is the one you create in your mind.' I sincerely believe in the truth of this statement. Share your findings with your child in a way that they can understand. For example, my daughter and I have a song that says, "I can do it." It's impressive to see the effect these few words have on her! You should never underestimate the ability of your child to understand principles such as these, even if you know their cognitive skills are impaired. Help them understand different concepts even if they cannot sustain a meaningful conversation with you about them.

Use a slow, steady, and methodical approach when working on your mindset. Take as much time as you need. The mind is delicate, and you must treat it as such. Use daily thought-starters by asking yourself a question. When a particular question and its answer are internalized and natural, that's when you'll know you've mastered that aspect of your mindset. The following is a list of thought-starter questions you can ask yourself:

- What is something new I can learn today?

- What did I do today that made me think about my decisions and actions?

- Have I worked on any challenges or problems today?

- Is there anything that made me feel stuck today?
- Is there another way to solve this complex challenge?
- Did I make any mistakes today?
- What lessons have I learned from those mistakes?
- Can I do something easy for myself today?
- How can I challenge myself with the same task even if it seems repetitive?
- What could I do better if I had the chance to learn how?
- Who can help me accomplish this?

This mindset shift shouldn't be limited to your child's needs. You can apply it to everything around you. It can involve communication with helpful people, building friendships, and relationships with other parents of special children. Let other people take care of your child when you're exhausted. Ask for help when you need it. Take a break when you feel overwhelmed.

Working on your mindset can be challenging, but it can become one of your greatest attributes as the parent of a child who is abled differently. The following are some tips to help you improve your mindset from negative thinking to positive.

Self-belief

When you believe in yourself leading the way, you are better equipped to interact with your child and deal with challenges, even when overwhelmed. Trusting yourself might take some time, but it's worth it. Moreover, when you trust your ability, the incidences of explosive emotions will reduce significantly. As a parent, you might feel stuck in the cycle and routines associated with caring for your child's needs. Often, this is communicated through emotional breakdowns, sadness, and the feeling of being overwhelmed. When you learn to trust your capabilities, these negative emotions decrease significantly.

Believing in yourself requires having clear goals. Work toward those goals using creative options such as bucket lists and vision boards, but don't pressure yourself. It's not a competition. Failure is part of the process. If you fail, you are not a failure; it just means you must recalibrate and get going again. Do not expect the path to be continually smooth. You may find yourself drifting back to your old ways of thinking. You might doubt your abilities and decisions even when you try not to. Address these setbacks immediately and determine what you can do to avoid repeating the same mistakes. You mustn't dictate every outcome; sometimes, you just have to let the universe unfold. Do whatever makes you feel comfortable, and take it one day at a time.

Success stories

Be inspired by other people's success stories. Reading real-life examples of people who struggled and overcame a negative mindset can be empowering. For instance, American-born Helen Keller lost her sight and hearing after a bout of illness at the age of 19 months. Despite enormous setbacks, she earned a bachelor's degree and became a prolific writer and disability rights advocate. Read her story and be inspired. You can find incredible stories online of the successes of people with disabilities and the sacrifice their parents often made to enable them to thrive. Reach out to them where possible, and you'll often find that they are accessible and willing to support you. Surround yourself with examples of people who persevered despite obstacles, including their failures, and succeeded.

We also have so much to learn from people outside of disability. Most people have heard of J. K. Rowling, who penned the famous Harry Potter series. Before anyone knew who J. K. Rowling was, several publishers rejected her manuscript multiple times. Yet, there was no giving up – she trusted her ability. She was confused and discouraged at times, but she persevered. Today, she is a respected author known worldwide for her fascinating work.

HARMONY

The environment also has a significant impact on your child's overall well-being. Children need a stable home and school setting to grow and learn. An unstable home can affect your child's emotional, intellectual, and social growth. Multiple studies reveal that when a child's surroundings lack harmony during their early years, their development may be impaired. They may end up with poor language skills, coping difficulties, behavioral issues, and challenges in school.

Furthermore, there are other long-term outcomes associated with instability. They include teen pregnancies, drug addiction, depression and anxiety, and suicide. Further studies on brain imaging show that a stressful environment permanently changes a child's brain development. This can impact other areas of the child's life, such as learning, memory, cognitive ability, and social and economic development. The stakes are even higher for children with special needs, who are often vulnerable and require additional assistance. For this reason, creating a harmonious school and home environment for your child is essential.

Intelligent children

One mistake I have witnessed parents of special children making is underestimating their child's intelligence. In my view, that's tantamount to child abuse. A child who is non-verbal is no less able to process the situation than a neurotypical child. The fact that they cannot articulate their thoughts verbally does not make them hurt any less. Always assume that your child is intelligent. They can tell when a situation makes them uncomfortable and react in their unique way. They take note of those squabbles in the home or disagreements with teachers or caregivers. I learned this early on when I witnessed my little girl crying when her dad and I raised our voices. We were not arguing, but our daughter thought we were. Years ago, we decided to avoid raising our voices, and our home has been far more peaceful for it. Please do not underestimate your children's awareness of what is happening around them. Pay attention and allow appropriate space for your child to speak into your home environment and shape it.

The emotional tone

Imagine walking with a colleague into a room full of people. They greet both of you warmly, smile, and make you feel welcome. You feel good because you know these people care that you came. Now, imagine that you both enter a room of people; they greet your colleague warmly but ignore you. Essentially they don't acknowledge your arrival, and you instantly feel unwelcome. The same applies to your special child when you discuss them rather than include them in their presence. You must acknowledge their presence and train others to do the same. Your child may have a disability, but their feelings are not disabled. Set the right emotional tone.

Create a harmonious environment at home that makes your child feel loved. Greet them with a smile in the morning, and when it's time to say goodbye, wish them a good day and hug them. When you are a caring, attentive, and positive parent, the home environment will reflect this. Remember to model this behavior in the presence of extended family and friends so that they behave inclusively to your child. Your child may be special, but they are a child first. Model positive behavior in public so that your child feels loved. It will build their esteem and confidence.

Consider adding pictures of familiar faces around the house to create a warm, homey space. Hang your child's drawings and artwork around the house where they can see it. Warm lighting and cozy materials such as blankets, pillows, and comfy chairs will give your home a sense of peace and serenity. Create a home environment that reflects every family member, including your special child and their favorite things.

Teachers and caregivers

You already know that taking care of and teaching a child with special needs takes more effort. I have seen many parents lashing out in the media about the school and medical system and how these systems are failing children. This might be true in your case, but it's not your fault, not your child's fault, not the teacher's or caregiver's fault. A teacher's job is to teach the curriculum in accordance with their training using the resources and within the constraints under which they operate. They are not medics or social workers. However, it's important to remember that they are probably not familiar with behavioral needs or neurodiverse behavior. Even if they are, they most likely only specialize in a particular field. You don't expect them to have all the answers; in reality, no one does.

I had a challenge some time ago with my daughter's primary school. They consistently complained about her behavior despite knowing that she had special needs. They had claimed to be an inclusive school and received additional funding to meet her needs. I wrote emails and had meetings, conversations, and other interactions but to no avail. I eventually had to invoke the local authorities, and we had a meeting of all the services involved and the school. We ultimately agreed that the school provision was unsuitable for my daughter, and she was withdrawn and allocated a space at a special school that suits her needs. At no point was there any hostility towards the school or the professionals, but I refused to allow my daughter to be stigmatized and ultimately traumatized. You have to know where to draw the line, bearing in mind that it's not what you do, but how you do it.

Many schools and institutions lack the funding and resources to help every child. The paperwork is overwhelming, and the bureaucracy is annoying. It might take weeks for something simple to be approved. Try to be patient, but stay in communication with your child's school to keep your child's needs in mind. This does not mean you should relax and not push for services for your child. Unfortunately, we live in a world where he who shouts the loudest gets what he wants. Advocate ferociously for your child but do so in a respectful manner. Treat all these parties as stakeholders in your child's life and try to secure win-win solutions to emerging problems.

Siblings and spouse

As a result of their additional needs, your special child can become your primary focus. You may be unintentionally ignoring other members of your household. Siblings and step-siblings of your special child must know they are loved and appreciated. You and your partner must also show them that you care for them. Don't forget that your spouse is also a member of the family who needs your attention. You probably have a hectic schedule, but this shouldn't be an excuse to neglect other family members. They need your attention too. Go on a date with your spouse or watch the latest movie together when your kids are in bed. Don't forget the popcorn! Have an ice cream or go window-shopping with your other children. Let everyone know they are loved and appreciated and are all important to you. Show them that you care about their needs and interests, and help them pursue and realize their dreams.

Your child is part of the family and needs to feel it. Family time imparts a sense of togetherness and responsibility within the home. Everyone in the family can create rules for a harmonious and peaceful existence. The rules should be presented positively, for example, "use a kind tone" instead of in a prohibitive way, "no yelling in the home."

Family time is an excellent opportunity for parents and children to develop ideas on resolving conflict around the house. Mealtimes, meetings, and project times are perfect bonding opportunities. Give your children time to discuss issues that are bothering them (and you!), and make some rules together that everyone can honor. By doing this, you help your children feel appreciated and included.

The role of nature

Nature adds beauty, a sense of harmony, and subtle creativity to our environment. Try to expose your child to the calmness of nature daily by going outdoors. The fresh air, natural environment, and your movement in them will significantly improve their physical and mental health, and yours too. Collect some items in nature and display them at home. Maybe your child loves seashells, rocks, plants, or interesting sticks—bring home whatever you can, and make a display to remember your fun day together. Your child will benefit from seeing your genuine appreciation for the great outdoors.

KEY POINTS OF CHAPTER 2

> Once you come to terms with your child's diagnosis and gather the resolve and hope needed to move forward, it's time for FAITH. You must be FEARLESS in taking ACTION to access appropriate resources, INVEST where necessary, and TRUST yourself to lead the process. Believe in yourself. Trust your ability to be there for your child and make sure you protect their interest. Finally, remember to maintain an environment of HARMONY at home, in school, and wherever you go, constantly circling back to the HEART of the matter—love for your child.

Chapter 3

PARTICIPATION:
The GENTLE Approach Solution

If you can't do it alone, do it together; and if you can't do it together, go it alone.
—Andrea Campbell

The GENTLE Approach Solution discusses the process by which one uses tools effectively to address your child's unique needs. It has chapters titled: **G**uidance, **E**njoyment, **N**urturing, **T**enacity, **L**earning and **E**mpowerment.

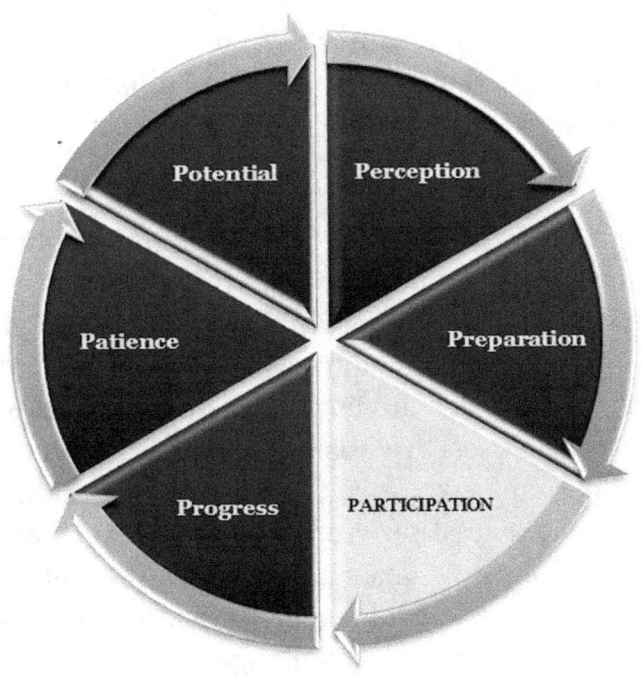

GUIDANCE

No one knows absolutely everything about a given subject. As parents of special children, in particular, we often find ourselves lacking knowledge or precedent, and yet the responsibility ultimately falls on us to care for our children and help them develop into their best possible selves. So do not be afraid to seek guidance. We often hear that knowledge is power; Albert Einstein once said: "Know where to find information and how to use it—that's the secret to success." So we must not only access information but also discern how to use it—in this lies our strength. First, however, we must find the available and appropriate resources.

Caring for a child with special needs can be an isolating experience. As your available time dwindles, your social network will likely follow suit, and your acquaintances and friends may disperse. This is not because they are bad people; it's just that your family's dynamics and demands have changed. Many of our children find it challenging to find and sustain friendships, and you must be creative to ensure they have a social life and do not get depressed or lonely.

If, as in my case, your child does not have siblings, there will be different demands on your time as often you must fulfill the role of your special child's household playmate. As a parent, especially, it's normal to feel isolated, but rest assured that you're not alone in this. At times you will likely wish that your closest friends and family could understand better and perhaps even speak about your situation, but this is an unfair expectation and might damage your most precious relationships. Instead, explore different platforms and social networks to find camaraderie and support related to your family's particular challenges. Many amateur and professional help and guidance are available to you when you reach out on the right platforms.

Assistance from parents and professionals

Parents of children with special needs form support groups that meet in their locale or online. Some invite guest speakers with specialist information that could shed light on your situation. A quick online search will reveal what's available. Find parent groups specific to your child's needs and reach out to members for help. These groups tend to be both focused and compassionate. They will not make you feel silly because they understand your journey. You can ask questions and expect to get answers explicitly related to your child's or family's situation. For example, I recently asked my group what I could use to treat my daughter's hair. She's on medication that damages her hair. Several group members replied with reasonable solutions. Some indicated that they had faced similar problems and told me what they had used. The given information proved helpful to me as well as other group members who might have the same problem. These groups are invaluable sources of support to parents.

Many parents have started blogs to share their experiences and teach others how to deal with the challenges of raising special kids. They are a source of inspiration and encouragement for parents. In addition, you can find people from all walks of life sharing their stories on social media platforms such as TikTok and YouTube. You may even be encouraged to start a channel of your own to share your story and inspire others.

In addition to parent groups, non-profit organizations provide advice that may be relevant to your child's diagnosis. While we cannot say that there is a support group for every medical condition, it is fair to say that there are groups for many conditions on the internet. Conduct a search and ask your school, doctor or social worker for help if you cannot find an appropriate one. This may be an opportunity to start a group if you cannot find one. If you are looking for learning resources and equipment information, you can ask professionals at your school for ideas.

You can also obtain information and guidance from books and specialist magazines. When looking online, be sure to check the source of information. The provider of information and advice should be reputable and preferably accredited, recognized in their respected fields. If you are seeking independent guidance, there are plenty of options, but be vigilant. Not everyone with an opinion is a professional, and not all advice will apply to your child. Take what works, and leave what doesn't.

Various magazines provide advice and guidance to parents of children with special needs. One such online magazine is the Complex Child E-Magazine, a free magazine written by parents dealing with challenges. This magazine gives you a platform if you've always dreamed of sharing your experiences. In addition, you are free to submit some of your work so others can learn from it. Complex Child has a vast database of information, and articles are arranged by topic so you can easily find what's relevant to you. You can also find links to organizations and support groups within your area.

Another good place to look for guidance is The Center for Parent Information and Resources (CPIR). It is an excellent place to find information on relevant products and services for children. If your child needs but is not yet isn't receiving home care, you can ask for guidance from home care providers. Some home care agencies function independently, while others are part of a larger entity.

The Exceptional Family Member Program serves military families with special needs. This program, administered through local support groups, has affordable housing projects and advocacy groups for when you need them. You can also find fantastic books, memoirs, biographies, and autobiographies online, some of which are free.

Further resources

Reach out for guidance and support from the many organizations willing to answer your questions and provide help when and support where necessary. Here's a list of support groups and organizations that are ready to help you:

Different Dreams - This organization describes itself as "a gathering place for parents of children with special needs" and provides parents with guidance, advice, and necessary support. They have a website with valuable resources and literature. In addition, multiple blogs on the platform highlight the challenges and joys of parents of children with special needs.

Mommies of Miracles - This organization reduces the isolation experienced by mothers of children with special needs. The organization provides guidance and an extensive network of resources for families of children with special needs. They support mothers when they need it. The platform welcomes mothers of children of all ages and needs. Some of the children have conditions that have not yet received diagnoses.

Family Monsters Project - If you are in the UK, Family Monsters is an organization that supports children with disabilities. They offer an EHC assessment that tests whether your child needs an education and healthcare plan. The goal is to highlight their educational and healthcare needs and provide support as necessary. The program caters to children and young adults from birth to age twenty-five.

Learning Disabilities Association of America - This website provides a comprehensive list of resources for parents, teachers, caregivers, and children with special needs families. They have an extensive list of competent organizations to get information about ADHD and learning disabilities.

National Parent Teacher Association - Their website offers tools for families, special education services in your state, and a list of national organizations you can contact.

You may also be able to find information and guidance from the American Academy of Pediatrics, Family Network on Disabilities and Enable Group. The official website of the US government is also a good resource.[4]

ENJOYMENT

Have you ever wondered how you could better help your child enjoy their time in the community? Your child is constantly going to therapy and attending appointments and school, but you can also create time for them to have fun. You can find activities they love, encourage participation,

---

[4] Visit https://www.ssa.gov/benefits/disability/ for information on government granted benefits for individuals with qualifying disabilities.

and reward them for achieving specific goals. The reward should be exciting and motivating. Remember that the things they love and enjoy should come first. Rewarding good behavior and progress help develop the child's language, behavior, and social skills. Let's discuss ways to help you and your child enjoy the journey.

Sources of Enjoyment

Play - You can use games your child enjoys to help them express themselves. Give them many intangible rewards—celebrate their wins and praise them simply for participating. Play therapy gives children an outlet and a sense of accomplishment, especially when they win. Then, involve other children in the games and show them how best to interact with their special sibling. Foster a sense of normalcy and let them understand that the child is just like them and shouldn't be treated differently.

Music - Simple repetitive words are easy to learn, especially in a song. They can also help a child with ASD improve their language skills. When the child matches their voice to the musical rhythms, they learn how to speak with more significant inflection—this is helpful for children who speak in a monotone manner. Music therapy is an excellent way for the family to enjoy time together. It promotes social interaction and can motivate a child to join in doing what they see their peers or family members doing.

Creative activities in the home - There are a host of activities that you, your special needs child, and your other children can do together. Try painting, reading, crafts, ball games, and threading. As a parent, I recognize that parents don't always have the time or desire to participate in the activities themselves. It can be overwhelming and exhausting;

sometimes, you wish the children would entertain themselves safely so you can get on with the chores or possibly even get a break. Where possible, enlist the services of a caregiver with the energy to keep your child engaged.

Personal interests - Show your child that you value them by paying attention to their interests. For example, is there a dish your child truly loves? What about a toy they've been obsessed with for a long time? Consider surprising them with one of their favorite toys. Scouting organizations offer an adaptable and structured framework for exploring interests at varying ability levels, and groups such as community theaters and recreation centers provide a supportive environment for specific skills. These interests may lead to a career or the development of new interests and relationships. For example, one parent in my local parents' group has a son with a keen interest in soccer. He learned the names of every club and the key players in the league. He was later able to volunteer at his favorite club and is well on his way to obtaining paid employment at the venue.

Community involvement - Children with disabilities are at high risk of social isolation, especially if they spend several hours a day confined to their homes or must attend weekly therapy sessions. Even if your child is non-verbal or has physical disabilities, it is not a good idea to focus on their disability and separate them from society. Instead, your goal should be to empower your children to be the best version of themselves. Help your child access activities such as swimming, bike riding, shopping, volunteering, craft fairs, holiday parades, museums, libraries, visits to friends, concerts, plays, parks, and playgrounds. As a result of their community involvement, they will develop and enhance their social skills.

Seasonal and sporadic activities - One way of having fun is embracing flexibility and adapting to daily life. For example, build a snowman or go sledding if it's snowing. If you've run out of your favorite cereal, make pancakes together. Join the library and spend an hour or two there. Sort the laundry and name the colors. If it's hot inside, go for a walk in a nearby park. By adapting to the available opportunities, you will find fascinating possibilities.

Self-Care

Focusing only on your child's happiness and not on your own would be unwise. Being a parent is demanding, whether or not your child has special needs. Please do not let this be the defining characteristic of your life. Parents are the primary caregivers, teachers, and nurses of their children. We accompany them through thick and thin, catering to their every need. The job can become all-consuming, and if we don't take care, we find ourselves so engrossed in caregiving that we ignore our personal needs. Do not let that happen. Remember that caring for yourself is also your responsibility. Anticipate situations and stress levels that will cause frustration. Make regular time for yourself. Here are some ideas:

Make new friends - You might connect more with parents in similar situations. Choose people with whom you have common interests and who refresh your spirit. Find friends interested in learning and with whom you can hold relevant conversations. Make sure you can connect on more levels than that of special needs struggles, though you may find it easier to relate to people who also have special children.

Learn a new hobby - A new hobby can keep your mind occupied when your child is away at school, in therapy, or with other caregivers and guardians. You can even become an advocate for your child and other children with similar needs. You can decide to be an expert in the field and advocate from an empowered position. You can also do other fun activities such as working out, cooking a new dish to surprise the whole family, spending time in nature, and planting a garden.

Relax - Don't overthink—overthinking robs you of momentary happiness. When you overthink, you anticipate the worst-case scenario. Hold the happy memories close and create new ones when you can. Don't let yourself become consumed by worry and sadness. Always look forward, never backward, because the life ahead is all you have. Don't become consumed by thoughts of what could have been and what-ifs.

Avoid negative people - Do you find some people always complain or have something negative to say? This includes healthcare practitioners, friends, relatives, and caregivers who always find something to moan about. If a doctor tells you that your child will never be able to do this or that, change them. Give them a break if your friends criticize you for not meeting up with them regularly. They are not bad people; they simply do not understand your journey. Protect your heart from people who want to weigh it down. You don't need drama; you need understanding, flexible people who appreciate, inspire, and empower you. Beware of hostile social media as well. Consider closing accounts if you find yourself emotionally drained by social media.

Practice gratitude - Be grateful for your family every day. There's a lot of good in life; our special children teach us this. As parents of these children, it is natural for us to worry about what this journey may bring because we face uncertainties about our capabilities, capacity, and the challenges that may await us. However, if we focus on what's working, we'll develop courage for the next phase of the journey. It takes little effort to be grateful for what we already enjoy in life. Of course, it's harder to be thankful for something that we didn't request or want. But we become more resilient when faced with life's biggest challenges and learn to overcome major struggles.

Maintain a positive mindset - A positive mindset is a skill that requires deliberate development. It rarely happens by accident. Learn to stay happy and enjoy the little things in life while being honest about your feelings. Instead of focusing on what might go wrong and how terrible that will be, concentrate on how you can turn things around to make things right again, should something negative happen. As a parent, you must prepare yourself for every possibility. However, shifting your outlook to perceive potential challenges as an opportunity rather than a threat or danger will help to cultivate a positive mindset.

NURTURING

In addition to fulfilling their basic needs, children need love, encouragement, and support. Children with special needs need even more of all three elements to help them develop a strong sense of self-worth and confidence. Parents must ensure that, as they focus on their children's cognitive and physical development, they are not ignoring their child's emotional development. Our job as parents is to help them see their self-worth and provide them with the appropriate social and emotional tools to help them learn. As a result, your child will grow stronger and more resilient as they approach adulthood.

The task of nurturing children with special needs can magnify if you are a single parent. However, it is possible to do it alone if you find the right attitude and balance your time appropriately between your child, work, and other commitments. You know your child best. You significantly impact their emotional, academic, social, physical, and overall success. If you nurture them in these areas, you will help them succeed to the best of their ability. You may need to specifically design your environment to meet a child's sensory needs and create the best setting to learn and achieve their potential.

Children with special needs will do best in a safe environment where they are free to express themselves with little consequences. While we want our children to relate to people, we must recognize that some children relate better to inanimate objects, like stuffed toys, where they can be free to express their emotions without criticism. Parents must manage the dynamics, allowing the children to have this outlet without building a wall around themselves. Let them feel empowered to be themselves while providing opportunities for interaction and building social skills.

The following are some tips for how you can create a nurturing, empowering environment for your child:

Keep things in perspective - Remember that everyone faces difficulties in life. Your child is not defined by systems or labels society might place on them. It may be difficult initially to deal with negative attitudes, but stay strong. Keep things in perspective by telling yourself that your special child needs you to model positive behavior in the face of life challenges. Also, find ways to receive encouragement. Ask someone to regularly remind you of your and your child's successes while being willing to listen and make you feel heard when you just need to rant about a failure. Keeping the bigger picture of your family's journey in mind will give you the strength to better model good behavior and help your child grow into a strong and confident adult. Remember that you have the most substantial influence over your child. They will follow the way you approach and do things. If you show your child that you are optimistic and confident, they will likely be able to approach life similarly.

Tap into their interests - Support your child in extracurricular activities they enjoy. Help them try new things and identify something they love and want to pursue long-term from these activities. Encourage them to embrace the challenges and always provide them with resources. As they follow their passions, introduce other activities such as learning about the sport or activity. You can help your child start a blog or vlog to share what they love, and you can search online for inspirational activities that encourage your child (and you) to participate locally and nationally.

Be mindful of your words - Children listen and understand every word from your mouth. When you say things like, "Tyler loves to throw tantrums", it becomes a self-fulfilling prophecy, the child internalizes the message and throws even more tantrums. It is better to rephrase the statement and say: "Tyler has a huge personality." Instead of reacting to his temper, suggest breathing exercises or quiet time until he calms down. When you use positive words, you nurture your child's innate abilities and send them a powerful message that they can accomplish anything if they put their heart into it.

Focus on their strengths - When we have children with special needs, we can easily focus on their disability rather than their abilities. Shift your attention to their strengths instead of their weaknesses. For example, my daughter struggles with motor skills and doesn't enjoy writing. She prefers to spell words and is particularly pleased when she gets them right. I, therefore, focus on her spelling and let her teachers concentrate on the writing. Some people don't like certain activities. No one is good at everything, so I have decided to focus on some things instead of others. You will know where to place your focus depending on what your child likes to do.

Acquire educational resources - There are myriad educational toys on the market. They allow the child to indulge in learner-led activities that make them happy. The Pocket Learner is one such resource. The child can use it independently or with siblings to cover many learning areas. This system supports a child's unique learning needs and abilities and presents information to the child in a new and different manner from what they might use at school. It is also a system that allows the child to show you what they can do and understand. Using the Pocket Learner educational resources and similar educational activities and toys will increase your child's confidence and excitement about learning.

Study the concept of neurodiversity - Neurodiversity might seem like a technical word, but it is pretty simple. It means the diversity of the human brain. The neurodiversity paradigm helps children with ASD and ADHD view the world in their unique way. They understand their way might differ from how neurotypical individuals view the world, but their method is entirely valid. It helps them consider their challenges as merely things they need help with simply because the world is designed for neurotypical brains. Help your child understand that this isn't necessarily bad. It's just the way it is.

Review the environment - Take a moment to consider your child's environment. Where do they spend most of their time? What's the nature of this environment? Is it calm or tense? Are there negative influences around the neighborhood? How is the school environment structured? Your child's environment can shape their behavior. You must try to provide a nurturing and stable environment for your child to the best of your ability. Observe them. Listen keenly. What can you see? What do you hear from the environment? Maybe all you need is a change. Sometimes a change brings encouragement and respite to the whole family.

Teaching and nurturing your special child often boils down to one principal goal–focusing on and building your child's strengths. Your child may have some difficulties doing certain things due to their disability, but they are not weak in all areas of life. Perhaps they are excellent at music. Encourage their talent in music and spend plenty of time nurturing that talent. The ultimate goal in educating a special child is to see them happy and content with life and able to excel as an adult.

Find out what works best for your child and persist in doing what you need to do for your child. For example, if your child has difficulty reading, help him by reading to him first. Then, approach the learning disability enthusiastically and show your child that learning at their own pace is okay. As time passes, your child will understand that it is ok to be slow as long as he is developing the necessary skillset.

TENACITY

Have you ever been told that you are a strong parent because you look after your special kid? How about "You are amazing; I don't know how you do it!" Yes, we are amazing, strong, fierce, determined, and creative parents navigating learning, attention, communication, and behavioral issues. Some of us care for children with complex medical needs–gastronomy tubes, seizures, neurological disorders, and dietary restrictions. Some of our children are in wheelchairs. We raise children with disabilities, but that does not make us saints. We show up every day and do what we have to do. We get up because we love our kids and want them to have a rich, meaningful life filled with joy and laughter. We get tired, overwhelmed, and worried in the process; platitudes such as those at the start of this paragraph can feel understated and pointless.

Parents of children with special needs worry more, work harder, deal with more systems, and live with more chaos. We often feel underappreciated, under-recognized, and frequently thought of as annoying or demanding parents. We have to learn to navigate medical, legal, and educational systems. You may find yourself policing your schools to implement your child's education plan, fighting your general practitioner to prescribe a particular medication or to refer you to a specialist. We've learned about occupational therapy, physiotherapy, and other therapies and treatments. We did not choose our life; it chose us, and most of us have risen to the occasion.

This kind of fight needs a higher level of tenacity. Demanding insurance to cover applied behavior analysis requires tenacity. Getting your child into a dance class in a wheelchair requires perseverance. Reminding educators that your child needs extra prompting can be very exhausting for parents who feel they must forge the way for their child in every aspect of life. Yet, you must stay the course if you want assistive technology support for your special child. When you're at the grocery store and your child gets overwhelmed, you must be strong to survive the stares and get yourself, your child, and your groceries home. It is not unusual for our special children to be left off the invitation list for birthday parties. You can't force people to invite your child, but you have to be creative to keep your child's spirits up in the face of discrimination. Your tenacity can turn to anger if your child receives teasing or bullying because of their difference.

Being a parent of a child with disabilities means we have more going on than parents of neurotypical kids. That doesn't make us better, but it makes our lives different, and just like our kids, the world is struggling to understand. You will hurt as you watch your friends leave and see your kids excluded. Focus instead on the new friends who understand your journey. Reach out to others who are on the same path as you are.

Keep hope alive

Having a special child can feel like an uphill climb, and some parents may feel the urge to surrender. Often it's not about a struggle with the child or the disability; instead, the many fights mentioned above require the most effort. It is easy to feel a sense of helplessness, inadequacy, and hopelessness. You may feel like you are letting down your kid, like you aren't doing enough. The many appointments, sessions, and meetings can be simply overwhelming. Everyone deals with issues differently, and it's okay to feel uncertain emotions but never let them get the better of you.

I have experienced fear. I have been overwhelmed. I have learned to take things one day at a time. I've accepted that some things are beyond my control. As long as I do my best, that is enough. What I do know is that I'll never quit. Be reminded that your child needs you, not only to provide for them but also to advocate for them. Despite feelings of inadequacy and frustration, you must keep on keeping on. Reach out to the people and institutions we discussed if you feel you need support. Sometimes we think we cannot keep going, and then we surprise ourselves and move into another gear. Where there's a will, there's a way. On some days, it will be challenging, and on others, it will be better. And there will be days filled with laughter.

If you need a break, take it. Tap into your support network or get help even if you have to pay for it. If you are too tired, you are more likely to make costly mistakes, so endeavor to take a break. Being a parent to a special child is just one part of your identity. Remember to nurture the other parts of your life. Change the plan if you get bored or realize that it needs modifications.

Never lose your sense of humor. Some things will get under your skin from time to time. Everyone has their issues. But if you aren't careful, you'll become so sensitive that people will avoid you altogether. Be cautious of the words you use in the presence of others. For example, phrases such as "I almost had a heart attack" or "It almost gave me a stroke" may sound insensitive to a parent whose child has suffered a stroke or a heart attack. If you are the parent of a child who has suffered this way, remember that the other person didn't say this to offend or upset you. They probably just said it as a common colloquialism with little extra thought.

Remember that you are not perfect and don't have to be. When you set the bar so high that you can't achieve it, you set yourself up for failure and the emotional roller coaster that may accompany it. Try to be realistic when setting goals. Adjusting plans to accommodate your child or the situation will propel things forward rather than trying to start from an unrealistic starting point. When you fail to achieve your goals, try to find the silver lining. If you maintain a positive attitude, you might discover that it was not as big of a loss or setback as you had thought. It helps to work on forgiving and embracing new chances.

Life is about hoping for a better tomorrow. We strive for what might be. If there is no hope, then what else is left? We must all strive for our children. We must fight to help them be their best selves and go as far as they can. Despite the challenges you may encounter, do what you need to do to stay the course. Take it one day at a time—be patient and keep a positive attitude.

Belief in your child's abilities

You've probably heard hundreds of stories about successful people who overcame huge setbacks because someone believed in them. This belief is often the defining factor in many success stories. That's not to say that you are the only person who believes in your child and is willing to do whatever it takes to help them succeed. The point is that sometimes it only takes one person to believe in you for you to believe in yourself; you can be that person for a child

When my daughter was eight years old, her teacher told us she should "just learn to make a sandwich." It was a painful moment for me, but I took that statement to heart and produced a set of resources to help my daughter learn and was able to help children across the globe. It says that if you can see beyond the negative comments and stay positive, you can create a good chapter in your story that positively impacts the lives of others.

Stick with your child through thick and thin. Stay by their side until they discover who they are and what they can do. Then, if circumstances are appropriate, continue to care for them. Your child is here for a reason, and you must believe it. The more support you give them, the better their chance to excel.

Tenacity pays off

The challenges of raising a differently-abled child can be frustrating but incredibly rewarding. Some situations can even be downright depressing. Yet there is always the chance that a breakthrough is just around the corner. You have invested love, time, and effort; there is no sense in giving up, ever. Instead, you must persevere with a determined spirit. If you raise a strong-willed child, the ultimate goal you could be giving the world is an unrelenting leader unswayed from what is right towards the mere popular.

Some parents have empowered their children to achieve feats even doctors believed they would never do. Rest assured that you will reap the rewards once you have the tenacity to keep going.

LEARNING

There's an old saying that teaching is a thankless job. Many teachers are underpaid, schools are understaffed, and some struggle to make ends meet. While teaching is demanding in and of itself, being the teacher of special children comes with an additional layer of challenges. Studies show that teachers of children with special needs suffer from high levels of burnout and a higher than average attrition rate. For this reason, your child may not get individualized attention at school. Your responsibility as a parent is to ensure your child is learning and to reinforce those areas that might prove challenging.

Every child is different, and a teacher is responsible for a class of twenty to thirty children. It would be helpful if every strategy were dedicated to a child's uniqueness and individuality, but this rarely happens because the teacher must teach within the curriculum and focus on the majority. In special schools, there is more individuality as children are usually in small clusters and grouped according to ability.

Learning isn't limited to academics. Children with special needs have gifts and talents that need nurturing. Some are artists, some are athletes, and others are entertainers. This is true for all children; your special child is no exception. As a parent, observe your child and ask yourself the following questions: Are they confident? What life skills do they have? What social and emotional skills do they have? Is there a way to nurture and build on what is already there? Can you find an effective way to bring a shy child out of their shell? Take every opportunity to foster learning. For instance, ask your child to bring you a blue cup, not just any cup. This allows them to consolidate their knowledge of colours. The following are strategies that you can use to encourage learning.

Put items out of reach - Your child may want certain things in the home - food, toys or essential items. Try putting these items out of the child's reach so they have to request them. If the child is tall, you may need to place the item in a space that is hard to access. If you are tempted to retrieve the item, you must resist that temptation. Instead, encourage the child to ask you for help to get the item. This will inspire them to communicate—to verbalize or use sign language to satisfy their needs and wants. This strategy is an excellent way to improve their social and communication skills.

Use chunking - Break down big tasks into small, manageable tasks. If you overwhelm the child, they will quickly lose motivation. Projects should be short, exciting, and engaging. If a project is complicated, it will confuse your child and lead to frustration. Complicating a task is counterproductive and reduces their willingness to complete it.

Clear communication - Make sure your instructions are straightforward enough for a young mind to comprehend. If the child doesn't understand an instruction, repeat it using more explicit language or examples to which they can relate. Give verbal prompts when necessary. When the child is non-verbal, use appropriate signs or body language to convey key messages.

Use charts and visual aids - Pictures, graphs, and charts drive the point home faster. Many children with learning difficulties respond well to visual stimulants. The Pocket Learner, for example, uses clear, colorful images that inspire children. These images appeal to children and enhance the natural interaction between the child and the parent/guardian/teacher during the learning process. This interaction builds their confidence and improves their social skills. The Pocket Learner also encourages using rewards to keep the children's attention and thus increase participation.

Frequent breaks - Some of our children have short attention spans. Learn to recognize the signs that they need a break.

Plan exercises that are easy yet somewhat challenging for your child. Then, when the child feels overwhelmed with learning, have them stand up, stretch, and do the exercises. You can also read them an exciting story or play a game. You can also converse casually with them about some of their favorite things. An opportunity to take a break can have a calming effect on the child.

Maintain a comfortable environment - Reduce or eliminate where possible environmental triggers. For example, some children are sensitive to loud noises, glowing lights, or temperatures that are too hot or too cold. These triggers can interrupt their thinking patterns and cause outbursts. Make it your business to know what triggers your child and try to avoid them. Unexpected or major changes in routine can have a significant impact on a child with special needs.

Create a predictable schedule - Predictable routines can be very beneficial. Make sure your child is familiar and comfortable with your routine. Letting the child set up the routine with you is one way to do that. This action will give them a sense of ownership, and they will be more likely to follow it. Tell them ahead of time, where possible, if something different will happen on a specific day. For example, if an emergency doctor's appointment is to take place or if someone else will watch them for a few hours, try to ensure your child knows in advance.

Create opportunities for social encounters - Children learn when they are around other children. Create fun projects for the kids and promote collaborative work. These projects can happen in small settings with friends and family or large settings such as a classroom. Create a positive, exciting experience for the kids to look forward to. The children should also participate in extracurricular events. Myriad activities may be possible, depending on where you live. Consider exploring nature, attending family fun fairs, or watching a movie. You can play indoor games, paint, or play with toys when it's cold outside. My daughter and I play catch the ball on the stairs in our house when the weather is unfavorable. It gives us a good workout.

Build on your child's strengths - Does your child love dinosaurs, dogs, or animals in general? Do they get excited when it's time for water sports? Are they obsessed with baseball or football? If you notice an interest in a particular subject, create opportunities for your child to showcase their expertise. Use the activities they love to promote learning. If your child is exceptionally talented in a specific activity, consider engaging a coach or other professional to help them hone their talent.

Teaching a child with special needs can be demanding, but if you are creative, you will find effective ways to teach and reinforce learning. Widen your perspective on learning to include academic, social, emotional, and independent learning strategies to enrich your child's educational experience. When children are involved with planning, they are happier to participate. Finally, reward your children for their hard work—this will give them a sense of pride and accomplishment.

EMPOWERMENT

You love your child and want to help them in every way possible. I know that because you are reading this book. It is a good thing to help your child, but how do you balance giving them the necessary support and empowering them to be independent without hindering their growth? Parents of special children navigate a fluctuating line between being there for their children and giving them space. We should be careful not to overprotect our children as they find their way in this world. Our job is to empower our children, build their confidence, and help them realize how much they can accomplish independently. Your child has special needs, but they are a child first. I avoid the term "special needs child" without exception; a child's special needs do not define them. Focus instead on empowering your child. Let's look at some ways to do so. Don't do everything for them. If the child can put on their clothes, make a sandwich, brush their hair or teeth—let them do it. Give them extra time if they need it, but let them do it themselves. It may be inside out or upside down but never mind; let them try. Then show them the right side up or help them part of the way and allow them to complete it. Always remember to praise and encourage them for their efforts. It may be easier at the moment to do things for them, but this doesn't empower them in the long run. Your patience will result in their gradual improvement.

Challenge them - Don't give them only easy tasks just because you want them to succeed. Instead, find jobs that require effort and practice to achieve. Lead the process by showing or working with them to complete the tasks. Then, if you want to observe their creativity, give them jobs and watch from a distance. Encourage them to ask for help if necessary. This very act of requesting will help their communication skills. When they work through challenges, the children soon understand that if they put their mind to something, they can achieve it with hard work. If you realize a task is too challenging for them, try to find ways to scaffold it down so that it is closer to their ability level. Once they complete the job, you can adjust it to make it more demanding. Try raising the level of difficulty but not to the point of frustration.

Give them choices - Providing choices is a simple but effective way to build a child's independence. Options give them opportunities to be in control of their lives. Giving them a choice shows them that you respect them and that they should expect others to respect them. Without overly complicating life, provide them with autonomy in their daily decisions. For example, ask them if they prefer a red or a black shirt, if they'd rather have an orange or a banana, or if they'd like to visit family or go to the mall. If they must do something less attractive, such as a dentist visit, let them decide who they would like to take them or pick a fun activity to do afterward. This also informs and prepares them. As you give your child choices, you slowly and consciously build their communication skills, self-esteem, and confidence to self-advocate. You may also earn yourself a bit of leverage for moments when you need your child to move along quickly under your guidance.

Set realistic goals - Sit down with your child and create a list of goals. Make sure to incorporate everything they are interested in and what they want to accomplish. Your child may be non-verbal, but body language and responses are a great way to include them. Goals motivate and incentivize them because they understand they are working towards something meaningful. Do your best to gauge where your child is at and set realistic goals. If you find a goal too tricky, apologize and simplify the task. Process your goal-adjusting out loud. "I thought you could make your teacher's card while I prepared dinner, but now I see that this project needs more time. I'm sorry for underestimating. Let's tidy up and finish together after dinner."

Remember that you are your child's best teacher; they will best learn the life skills needed to navigate life with or without a disability from your modeling. This will help your children learn to work with you. It will also help them learn to forgive themselves as they gauge their readiness and revisit hopes and goals. Make use of assistive technology. We live in a time when technology is constantly advancing. For example, we can now instruct our televisions to turn on or tell our device what song to play without lifting a finger. Let your child participate in the information technology revolution by using communication devices, special switches, buttons, utensils—any useful implements that make their life easier as they navigate independently.

Work with teachers and therapists - Work with your child's teachers and professionals to create consistency in building independence. Clear and honest communication as you share tips and strategies will help your child grow. Together you will discover what works and doesn't and needs to change. Transparency will help your child develop self-awareness and take increasing ownership of the challenges they must face.

Safety first, but only where necessary - As a parent or guardian, our first job is to keep our children healthy and safe. Sometimes, however, we wrongly gauge what our children can handle. Naturally, you are tempted to "save" your child from a stressful situation even when no danger is involved. Wherever possible, let your child navigate the problem on their own. The gift of independence is truly priceless. Your standing back will reassure them that you believe in them. It will also teach them that struggling is normal; they will understand that they can handle the challenge and grow in resilience. It may be painful to watch them struggle alone, but imagine the feeling you'll get when they can finally brush their hair, make a sandwich, or read a book.

KEY POINTS OF CHAPTER 3

> The GENTLE approach will empower your child with the social and emotional tools they need to deal with life's challenges. Seek GUIDANCE from recommended professionals and resources. Find ways to make your journey together ENJOYABLE. NURTURE your child's unique gifting. Remember, your child's special needs are only one aspect of their personality. Seek out and provide opportunities for them to develop their talents and shine. Exercise and model TENACITY. Always be on the watch for LEARNING opportunities. EMPOWER your child to learn new skills and take ownership of their development wherever possible.

Chapter 4

PROGRESS:
The JOY Generator Blueprint

The road to success is dogged by urges to quit. Don't let the dogs out!

—Andrea Campbell

The JOY Generator Toolkit uses consistent monitoring and evaluation to propel forward motion and create space to celebrate achievements during the process. We will work through **J**ubilation, **O**pportunity, and **Y**ield.

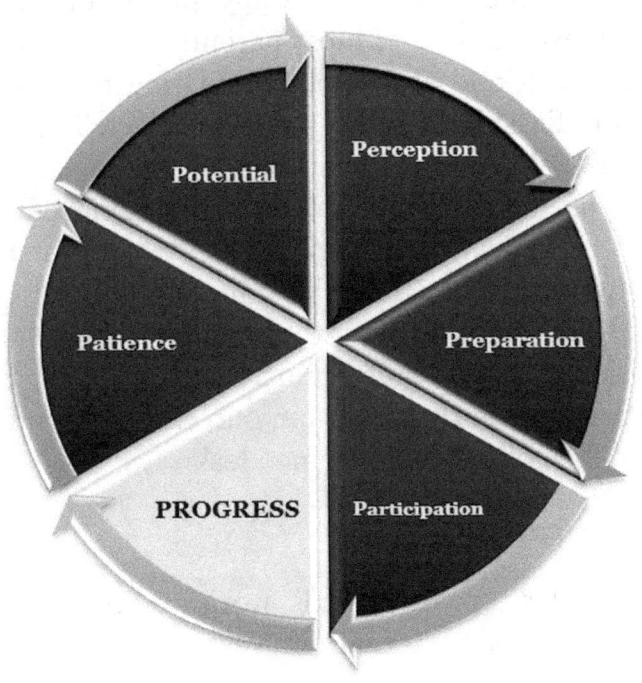

Jubilation

Most people welcome words of praise, even as adults. Everyone loves a few moments of appreciation following an achievement. Children love being appreciated too, especially by their parents. There are lots of accomplishments you can celebrate with your child. You can celebrate small victories like having eaten all their vegetables at dinner, sat for five minutes, or completed a two-minute task. You can also celebrate more significant steps: maybe they have gained an award, started a new hobby, joined a sports club or created a piece of art. There is a saying in the Caribbean: encouragement sweetens labor. When we show appreciation for our children's efforts, they perform better.

A study done by Greatschools.org on fifth and sixth-grade children with learning disabilities revealed some interesting facts (Kim-Kregal, 2011). When they asked the children what they were incredibly proud of, they listed specific achievements that most parents overlooked, such as making a new friend at school, completing their homework on time, and finishing a social studies project. The study also showed that children with special needs genuinely value social and academic achievements. Such achievements may not come as quickly to them as they do to neurotypical children, which makes the achievement a greater cause for jubilation. Let's look at how these small achievements can become more significant gains. Our job is to show appreciation and enthusiasm for our children's efforts and successes. The following are some ideas.

Generous Praise

An adage states, "praise words work." You may also be familiar with the alternative version: "encouragement sweetens labor." Those are factual statements. Words of praise are meaningful for adults but even more critical for children. Phrases such as "good girl, well done, excellent job, great stuff" will significantly impact your child's morale. Praises aren't just limited to words, however. You can incorporate physical gestures such as hugs, enthusiastic thumbs-ups, and high-fives.

The Pocket Learner is particularly keen on the element of rewards, including intangible ones such as praise. When children feel appreciated and know someone has noticed their efforts, they are motivated to do more. Eventually, they develop skills in that area because they love doing it and associate it with praise. For example, let's say your child doesn't like washing his hair. Praise them for their efforts and give them a high-five whenever they wash their hair. Use specific praise, "I love this blue part of your picture; it makes me think of the wind blowing through my hair." or, "You ate your food so carefully today; we didn't even need to wipe the table!"

Some children have high expectations of themselves and can become frustrated when they receive praise for something they feel they should be able to do anyway. Sometimes it is helpful to deal out moderate but very heartfelt praise, "I know that's not always been easy for you, but you gave it another go. I'm proud of you." Others thrive on the recognition and celebratory spirit of words of praise with each step that they take. You must gauge what works best for your child.

Display their achievements - Displaying your child's accomplishments is an excellent way to show them their achievements are worthy of recognition. You don't have to spend a lot on this. You can use simple frames to display their certificates, graduation pictures, art pieces, and more. You can get the certificate laminated or, at the very least, place it in plastic pockets. You can rotate the displays to make sure you highlight all significant moments. You can also hang small displays on refrigerators or a small bulletin board. Perhaps the easiest method is to hang a line of twine on a wall and use clothespins to secure the display. Sometimes your child creates impressive art and craft pieces, some of which are so good that they become treasures that last a lifetime. One way to inspire your children and show appreciation for their work is to display the art with labeled tags bearing their names.

Design a visual reward system - Make a visual display of your child's goals. Motivational stickers are a favorite for many parents. Child psychologists agree that sticker charts are fun, excellent ways to reward children for their achievements and good behavior at school and home. Consider also putting a puzzle on a bulletin board; your child gets a puzzle piece for each success.

Give physical rewards - Along with intangible rewards you can give the child physical rewards. Figure out your child's currency—it may be a toy, screen time, money to save for something bigger, or a treat to eat. Save these rewards for tasks requiring your child to get uncomfortable or work hard to move forward. Appreciation is most effective when done promptly. Give the physical gift immediately whenever possible. Some children like to choose a small prize from a basket; others do better when a specific reward is agreed upon and placed on top of, for example, the refrigerator for them to look at and keep in mind as they work on their chart to receive it.

Treats and experiences are also valid forms of affirmation. Create a chart at home, and keep it simple. List goals the child hopes to achieve with a treat of their choice. This should be something they enjoy and look forward to, such as a movie, a family picnic, playing in the park, getting a new book, getting an item with one of their superheroes on it, or going to a theme park. You can also present treats and experiences as "celebrations," including the whole family or friends. When planning a complicated project your child must tackle, it can help to include a celebratory treat once the task ends. The entire family will be proud of them, and the children will be delighted.

OPPORTUNITY

Children are natural explorers and learners, no matter their ability. They love fun, engaging activities that stimulate their brains. Take advantage of every opportunity to show them something new and engage their brains. This activity isn't just academic; it also embodies learning through play and the opportunity to discover. Let them play, and don't always feel you need to supervise or be an umpire. Children are creative whether playing with other children or by themselves. If they want you to participate, they will come looking for you. There are times when you are the leader and times when you are the follower. There are countless places where children can learn. Make it a habit to identify lurking opportunities and maximize your child's learning chances. The following are some ideas to keep in your back pocket. As a parent, you should know which activities are appropriate for your child as some may not be apt for every child. The guidance here is to identify opportunities for your child to learn, adapt them as necessary, and always be present to inspire, protect and empower.

Discover the kitchen - Most children love to help prepare food and learn a lot in the process. Give them light tasks such as picking the ingredients, washing them, and stirring them together in a bowl. Depending on their age and interest, you can let them help or give them a spoon and plastic bowl to mimic your actions. As they help, you can let them name the different ingredients. You can tell them stories and fun facts about the ingredients—their origins, nutritional value, and medicinal uses. Children love exciting stories and fun facts because they remember stories they hear. Some people choose a lower drawer in the kitchen and fill it with kitchen items that are safe for their children's exploration. Give it a label and explain to your child that it is their special drawer. Teach them to tidy up their "work area" as well.

Read books together - Find a comfortable position for you and the child and settle in for a story time and a cuddle if your child wants it. Read exciting books and ask for their guesses and input about the storyline. Pull out family photo albums and let them identify familiar faces. Teach them the names of family members, some of whom they might not know. You can also teach them about your ancestry and genealogy. Tell them stories of family members who are no longer with you. Do they know who their great grandparents were? Can they name their grandparents? Do they know all their cousins? What about their uncles and aunts? Are they in the same country, or do they live elsewhere?

Make videos - Create videos of all the fun activities you do together. Play the videos and laugh about them together. You can also record audio as they read, sing, or laugh and play it for them later. Playback the singing and laughing sometimes; have fun listening to it and looking back at the happy memories.

Search street and shop signs - Let the child read and count as you are out and about. They can read road signs, shop signs, or the signs on parks and buildings. They can identify different colors or count items such as cars and shops on the streets. When they recall a color correctly, you can give them a high-five. You can also count along with them and correct them gently when they miss a number. I've found that this activity is an excellent opportunity to learn and a fun bonding experience for parent and child.

Play learning games - Learning in motion is an excellent way to stimulate your child's brain. You can start with games that help them identify shapes and colors or learn about farm animals. For example, you can play a scavenger hunt where the child searches for different colors. Turn this into the game, I spy. If the child is a little older and willing, you can adapt these games to other areas such as history, foreign languages, anatomy, math, and earth science. Your imagination is the limit when it comes to learning games.

Listen to and produce music - You can use a wide range of music and musical activities to inculcate a love for music in your child. Add creativity and imagination by making your own instruments using household trash. For example, my daughter enjoys using a spoon to drum on a plastic plate. This is another excellent use for the items in their special kitchen drawer. You can also record instrument sounds together and then play them another day to see if the child can identify the sounds. It is easy to download simple recording applications on a smartphone. Next, acquire an instrument and work towards your child being able to handle it to do some musical exploration. Don't rush to make this an unsupervised activity—enjoy time together on the instrument. Another idea is to create a music trivia game where both find and cut out the answers from old magazines and newspapers. All this depends on the child's capability; you must choose which ones are suited for your child and adapt as necessary as there is something for everyone.

Complete homemade science experiments - When you think of science experiments, you probably imagine massive explosions that are wild and dangerous. It doesn't have to be this way. You don't have to turn the house into a blast zone to teach your kids science. Instead, you can do simple, safe experiments that fascinate your child and feed their curious nature. One experiment we perform at home is the homemade lava lamp. For this experiment, you will need an effervescent tablet (such as Alka Seltzer), a clear glass, one-quarter full of water, and a few drops of food coloring. Add double the amount of vegetable oil as water, so the glass is now three-quarters full. Drop the tablet into the liquid and watch the bubbles oozing. Add a light source such as a flashlight to the bottom of the glass for added effect. The lessons to be learned from this experiment are:

1) The water and the oil did not mix (because water is denser than the oil, so it sits at the bottom of the glass)

2) When the tablet drops into the bottle, it dives to the bottom and dissolves, creating carbon dioxide, which (like the oil) is lighter than water, thus causing bubbles that rise to the top and explode on the surface. After that mini-explosion, the colored water returns to the bottom, creating an oozing, lava-like effect in the bottle.

3) After a storm, there is a calm

4) Not everything that's combined mixes well (people included)

5) Everything naturally returns to a state in which it is comfortable.

Those lessons went beyond science but don't be afraid to stretch the teaching, depending on what your child can absorb.

Enjoy gardening - Tending the garden is more than sticking a seed in the ground and waiting for it to grow. Gardening provides opportunities for lessons in patience, science, and nutrition. Gardening teaches young children how plants come to life. It teaches them the value of life and what it means to care for something. Children also tend to be more excited about eating something they planted and cared for themselves. Perhaps the child can keep a gardening journal. They can record the plant's scientific name, nutritional value, and recipes used. They can also monitor the plant's growth and how long it takes before it is ready for harvest. If the plant is edible, everyone can taste what the child planted and let them bask in the glory of being a budding farmer.

The world around your child is full of learning opportunities. Teach them to curiously engage in their world, learn from it, and enjoy their discoveries.

YIELD

The formal education system requires parents to be flexible, understanding, and patient. Your child is one of many whose needs educators must address. Always approach educators with a grateful and appreciative attitude. As parents or guardians, you will collaborate with educators and the school, but you can also take an active role in documenting and monitoring your child's progress. You can do so much as a parent to plot a route for your child actively and have meaningful conversations with educators about your child's learning progress.

The importance of measuring

Good recordkeeping is key. Without proper analysis and documentation, you'll have no way to objectively and accurately track your child's progress, strengths, and areas for improvement. Keeping written records makes it easier to create a strategy to work on areas in which they are weak. Your child's learning progress is constantly under the lens at school through tests, assignments, quizzes, observations, and projects. In my experience, children with special needs have less homework, but they do have some. If your child cannot tell you, find out from teachers what lessons are being taught at school and find a way to mirror these at home. Communication with busy teachers can be challenging; many parents fear their children may be behind in their learning.

Tracking progress - To allay these fears, take positive action when you notice that your child isn't meeting expectations. Talk to teachers about their methods, seating arrangements, duration of lessons, or any other aspect of teaching that might have been overlooked. Work with educators to change whatever is not working and set goals for your success with your child. Most parents aren't aware of the abundance of technological developments available to them and their children. They are constantly changing, so this is understandable. Don't be afraid to ask outside sources, but keep in touch with your child's teacher and school as they will have the best idea of what your child needs. Many schools use innovative platforms with in-app portals for parents who want to be included. These are designed with integrated trackers that summarize a child's learning progress based on their level of engagement. If you are uncertain about something you see, be sure to ask your child's teacher. These platforms are limited in their ability to scaffold for different needs and can often be frustrating for students who perform at different levels. The Pocket Learner is also an excellent tool to track progress at home and in school.

Social progress - Parents want the best for their children. Academic performance is good, no doubt, but you should also find non-academic learning experiences for your child. You can also track their social progress. Do you know your kid's friends? Get to know them and connect with their parents if possible. You can also help to support your child's relationships with their friends. You must also consider the influence those friends have on your child. Encourage your child to seek out positive friends and associate with kids who avoid trouble and aspire to improve themselves. As your child becomes a teenager, their social progress becomes even more critical. Always try your best to monitor both social and academic progress equally. Whatever actions you undertake in the community or at school could have a spin-off benefit to your child. Following are several ideas to enhance your contribution to your child's progress at school.

Open communication - It will be tough, impossible even, to monitor your child's progress if you are unwilling to coordinate with teachers and other professionals. This can be done through phone calls, texts, or emails. You'll find those professionals eager to help and see progress, just as you are. Doctors, therapists, teachers, and everyone involved in your child's life are interested in your child's progress. Don't be afraid to express your concerns to the relevant professional.

Volunteer at school - There are many compelling reasons why a parent would decide to volunteer at their child's school. First, volunteering at your child's school is an excellent way to show that you are interested in their education and progress. Your presence around the school motivates the child to do better, and it's an excellent way to monitor their academic progress while helping the school with other duties. Some children love to see their parents at school, especially when certain events occur, but you always want to assess how your child feels about your presence there and whether visiting you in school makes them uncomfortable. If the child seems embarrassed with you taking an active role, you can do volunteer activities behind the scenes. Ensure the child understands that you are not spying on them but only trying to help the school.

In some cases, like mine, visible parental volunteering at school can be a deficit for a child. My child would cling to me, which would not be good. Some children need school to be their own space.

Keep going - This is probably the most crucial thing in monitoring and documenting your child's progress. Never give up on them, even when it looks like you've given it your all and they are still not making significant progress socially and academically. Speak with teachers and other professionals, and look at possible adjustments you can make. They can't guarantee improvement, but they can make genuine attempts to help your child.

Your role as a parent or guardian isn't limited to strategic, financial, or emotional assistance. You are a key person in your child's life, and you significantly influence your child's social and academic progress. Therefore, you must try your best to monitor your child's holistic development. Your guidance in their learning and growth process will be your best investment in their future.

KEY POINTS OF CHAPTER 4

> Many people assume that the lives of families with children who are abled differently are less happy because of their special needs. This misconception couldn't be further from the truth. Families of children with special needs are blessed. Your child brings joy and happiness to your family. Your life is more hectic, but taking care of a child with special needs teaches you how to see life differently. Find ways to celebrate your child's and family's progress in JUBILATION. Take every OPPORTUNITY you have to support your child's learning and encourage their curiosity. Monitor and track your child's YIELD using the platforms provided by your child's school to keep in close communication with their teachers.

Chapter 5

PATIENCE:
The LOVE Game Strategy

If you find yourself without, go find yourself within.
—Andrea Campbell

The LOVE Game Strategy describes the attributes required for developing staying power. It covers: **L**istening, **O**riginality, **V**ocalization and **E**ncouragement.

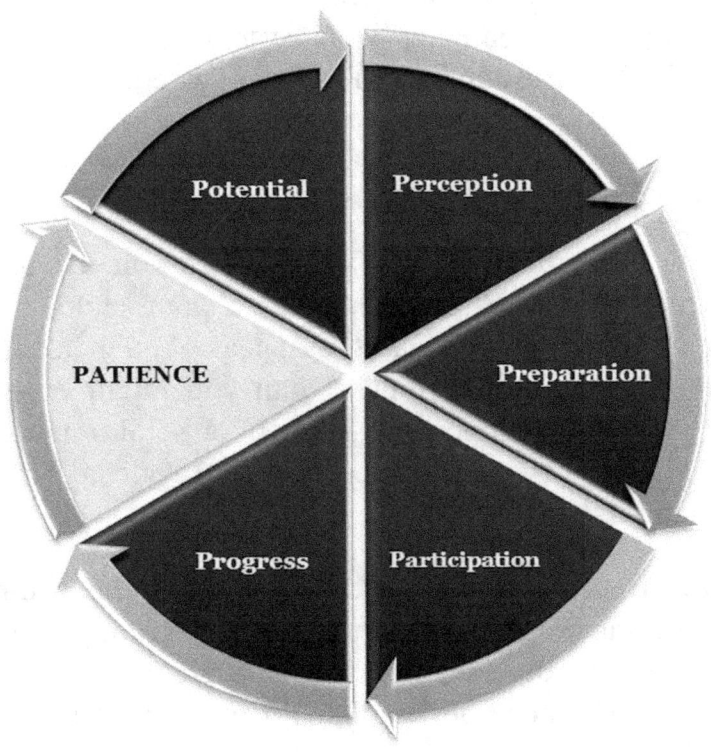

LISTENING

Listening is one of the most significant elements of being the parent or guardian of a child with special needs. Your patience will be tested because sometimes you will have to wait a long time to see your child progress. A child is more likely to listen to their parents if the parent listens to them. Isn't this what most parents want? When you listen, your child is more likely to do the same, and when they feel understood, they are likely to understand your point of view. Listening helps you and the child form stronger bonds, create better relationships, and build self-confidence.

Listening isn't just an externally directed activity. It is also essential to listen to ourselves—what do you want? Listen to your gut instincts and your body. This form of listening also means controlling your emotions, noticing your body, and changing your system if your intuition dictates it. If, for example, you're feeling tired, arrange some respite.

The importance of listening

Listening strengthens a child's bond with you. It increases their trust in you. While talking with your child, make a conscious effort to listen as they speak. You'll need to be patient if it takes them longer than you might expect for them to say what's important. Many of our children are non-verbal or may have some speech but struggle to articulate their thoughts effectively.

Nevertheless, encourage them to share their thoughts and emotions with you by prompting them and modeling good practice. Be sensitive and understanding in your responses, whether they say positive or negative things.

Before correcting what they say, intentionally acknowledge or repeat what they said to feel heard and understood. Also, check your response. Remember that your body language, facial expression, and tone of voice often speak even louder than your words. Are you communicating that you value and respect what your child has said? Or are you simply waiting for your turn to correct and teach them? Finally, think about how you want people to respond when you share something, especially if you share vulnerable emotions or frustrations.

In the case of children with limited speech or who cannot articulate verbally, you will need to 'listen' to their body language. Parents indeed know their children best. Health professionals and caregivers ask questions about your child because you are the expert on how your child behaves and reacts to situations. So understand that you must learn to "read" and listen to your non-verbal child because they have language.

Listening is not necessarily a straightforward process. You may be tempted to raise your voice and shut down the child when they say something with which you disagree. It might take extraordinary patience to listen to your child, especially when they say something that challenges your views, beliefs, and opinions. Some kids are naturally outspoken about everything they feel, whereas others require encouragement to speak up. For example, some children with high functioning autism may utter socially unacceptable words. What they regard as honest observations can be viewed as insensitive mutterings to the receiver. Your presence and carefully weighed responses can ease unintended tension in the situation. You may find it appropriate to apologize in a way that does not make your child feel undermined or belittled.

In listening to your child, pay attention to unspoken words. Our children are often misunderstood and written off as ornery when in fact, they are experiencing one or more issues. They may be in pain, experiencing gastrointestinal problems, food allergies, hormone imbalance, side effects from medication, endocrine disorders, or vitamin deficiencies.[5] This is not an exhaustive list; the lesson here is: don't be too quick to draw conclusions about negative behavior in your child—use all your senses and listen to your gut as you care for your child.

The role of empathy

The goal shouldn't be to respond to everything your child says. Instead, listen to what they want, what they'd like to do, and how they'd like you to help. Consider how you felt as a child. Is there anything you wanted the adults around you to do differently? Think of those times when you had so much going through your mind and wanted to be understood, but you just didn't have the right words. Put yourself in your child's position and do what you'd have wanted an adult in your life to have done. Listen without judgment and try to understand.

When you're empathetic, you don't judge, blame or criticize. Even if your child does not have the skills to respond to you, they can feel insulted or verbally abused. Don't shut them down in anger; instead, put yourself into their shoes and be understanding. Remember that this is your special child; you are on the same team. This is

---

[5] Often our children's non-verbal behavior is their way of trying to communicate a physical problem. Visit https://tacanow.org/family-resources/medical-causes-of-aggression-in-autism/ for some examples of ways that behavior can be a form of communication.

teamwork, not a competition. Many ways are more effective than yelling, sarcasm, or belittling to make a point. Lecturing is an excellent example of imposing yourself and your views on the child. Lecturing is about your opinions and making sure they are understood. You should refrain from lectures, especially with a sensitive child. If you choose this route, the child may shut you out altogether and cease to talk with you, even when they have serious problems. Instead, try to engage in meaningful, balanced conversations that foster independent thinking and sensible conclusions; you'll both be happier.

Some parents argue that children are too young to give constructive feedback. This notion couldn't be further from the truth. When I was a child, there was a common saying that "children must be seen and not heard." The irony is that children with a cognitive disability would never conform to that demand. They make intermittent noises, and it is very little we parents can do about it. Children observe and understand a lot of what we say, even if they cannot respond. They always think of what made you speak or act a certain way. Help them understand by encouraging them to communicate.

Practice active listening

When you listen to the child, demonstrate to them that you expect feedback and welcome their opinion. In these cases, a dialogue is better than a monologue. To encourage participation, you can even ask them how they feel about some of your actions. For example, a parent in our support group explained that she increases engagement with her daughter (who is autistic) by asking her, "What's the plan?" The child sees this as a cue to share her views on the situation.

Listening actively will help you get down on the same level as your child and sit beside them or engage a bit in their activity to express that you are on their side, not trying to control them or nullify their feelings. Sitting opposite them, or at a higher level, gives some sense of you being in charge, which may not be interpreted well by the child. Observe your child and listen to what they love to do. Support them or ask if there is a way you can help them. Keep your voice, attitude, and body language in check, even when you disagree. When they finish talking, ask why they think that is the right thing to do or say. If their reasoning is sound, let them be.

The whole point of listening is to understand your child's perspective. Maintain a calm tone. If you raise your voice with your child, they will probably increase their tone. The escalation may cause them to feel scared and stop talking altogether. Always try to de-escalate a situation by speaking with a calm, firm, controlled tone when necessary. If you get out of control and raise your voice, apologize to your child and admit that you are working on being a better listener. You both may need some time to cool down a bit.

It is important to note that when you encourage conversation with your child, you teach them to communicate effectively, negotiate, and problem solve. In addition, you are building their confidence—these essential skills will help them through life.

ORIGINALITY

Every child is different. Even identical twins are unique. A child's individuality emanates from two main factors: the child's genotype or nature, what they are born with, and the environment in which they live. Thus, even if twins have a similar genetic code, although they are still likely to be quite different, they will each interact with the environment in their unique way. No two children are the same. They might resemble you, your partner, their siblings, or other relatives, but apart from this, they have distinct traits that differentiate them from everyone else, from birth through adulthood.

Your child is unique. As you care for your special child, you learn their peculiarities, personalities, likes, dislikes, dreams, goals, talents, sense of humor, creativity, and gifts. Nature and nurture work together to shape a child's uniqueness. A child may be talented in certain areas. Still, support and affirmation from parents and people around them will likely encourage them to choose activities they love, thereby developing their talents and capabilities. For this reason, parents must find out what their child's talent is and build on it.

Sadly, some parents don't realize this, at least not soon enough. They have preconceived notions about what they want the child to be when they grow up and expect them to act in a specific way. For example, some parents wish their kids to be friendly, curious, quick learners, energetic, easy-going, and liked by everyone, among other "desirable" characteristics. When the child doesn't show the traits they expect, they experience disappointment. They feel like the child doesn't meet their expectations and grieve this loss. If a child senses that they have disappointed their parent or guardian, they will inevitably become discouraged or frustrated and respond negatively to the parents. A child who feels like a disappointment to their parents may struggle with anxiety, feelings of being unworthy, low self-esteem, and low self-confidence, and they're more likely to develop defiant behavior.

Developmental disabilities are a common obstacle in building a positive parent-child relationship. But suppose that you can look beyond a child's disabilities and value them as unique individuals as a parent. You can affirm and encourage them while providing the necessary support for their challenges. Your child will be in an excellent position to grow and progress when you do. Your encouragement and support will foster self-acceptance and natural resilience in children.

When you recognize your child's uniqueness and love and accept them for who they are without conditions, you will be better positioned to get through the inevitable difficult times. These difficult times make celebrating the good times together all the sweeter. The following are some ideas for celebrating your child's uniqueness, knowing them better, and providing them with the encouragement they need.

Discover - Observe your child daily, up close and from a distance. Note any changes in their behavior, physical appearance, emotions, and habits. Be attentive to new skills and new interests they might be developing. Interact with your child and experience their uniqueness by spending time with them.

Exposure - Take your child to every available opportunity to try new activities. You can visit museums, beaches, nature parks, and zoos. You can look for opportunities to explore sports, drama, art, music, reading, painting, fashion, movies, and a plethora of activities. Encourage them to try these things, and pay attention to the activities that make them light up. If they discover something they love, support them in it and encourage them to give that hobby their very best.

Conversion - If they want to quit, ask them why they want to give up. Encourage your child and let them know that they must push harder, even when tasks are tedious or challenging, but don't make them do something they no longer enjoy. At some point, you might have to let them quit if they want to. You might think they can succeed in a particular area, but you should never impose yourself on them. If you've exhausted all options and want to quit, let them do it without trouble. It is not unheard of for children to return to the activity when they are ready. They may not be able to express their feelings, so let them determine the timing for some activities. My daughter used to dislike swings. She would not go near them for several years. I was pleasantly surprised, however, to see her happily swinging during a recent visit to the local park.

Observation - This is the most exciting part about being a parent. It's okay to sit back, relax, and let your child be. Maybe they're playing a game, performing in front of a crowd, showing off something they are good at, playing an instrument, attempting comedy, playing at a tournament, and drawing—no matter what the activity is, watch, enjoy, and laugh with them! Celebrate with a smile, a hug, a high-five, and be there to praise and encourage them. Be their biggest cheerleader. You can take pictures or videos to capture the memories and relive those moments later. These are fantastic opportunities to spend time together and bond.

VOCALIZATION

Child experts say that vocalization skills can help a child build platonic or romantic relationships at school or work and even grow in self-awareness. You can encourage your child to speak and communicate in some gentle ways.

Training your child to be vocal is an essential life skill that will help them in the future.

Take every opportunity to encourage your child to vocalize, especially if the child has a speech delay or impediment or if they lack confidence. Ultimately, teaching your child to vocalize, or to use hand signs to communicate if they are non-verbal, will help them in all areas of their lives. Being able to vocalize will help them immensely in self-advocating. Whether learning to say no when they don't want to do something or speaking up when they have something important to share, assertiveness gives your child the strength to make sure they are heard. It builds their self-confidence. The following suggestions will help your child with vocalization skills so they are empowered to share their opinions wherever they are.

The role of questioning

Let them answer for themselves - Whether your child is greeting a friend or ordering a meal at a restaurant, let them speak independently. This also applies to non-verbal kids. Encourage them to use sign language, a communication app, or other media to convey their wants and needs. Many parents want to make their children's lives easier and "help" them in such situations. They are happy to encourage conversation in the home but less inclined to do the same in public. Remember that your special child is valuable to society and view these encounters as an opportunity. Let your child speak for themselves. You'll be amazed when they do, and you'll both feel that the child's opinion is valued and imperative in the situation.

Create time for interactive discussions - Make time each day to conduct meaningful conversations with your children and the whole family. For example, you can talk during meals or when you are out taking a walk together. Talk to each child about meaningful things and ask their opinions. Let them answer. Show them that you are genuinely curious about their thoughts.

Asking questions - asking your child questions is a good way of encouraging your children to vocalize. 'How' and 'why' questions will generate more in-depth answers. For example, the question: "What are your thoughts on this?" requires the child to explain their thinking process regarding a particular situation. Other questions you could ask include:

- How did you come up with that opinion?
- How did you learn that?
- Would you do things differently?
- That sounds interesting. Tell me more.
- Would you like to share more about that?

Don't end conversations with, "Ok." Instead, encourage your child to share more on the subject. You can use phrases such as, "I wonder why" or "How did that happen?" Such terms allow your child to think, talk, and share opinions.

Give them choices - I have already discussed the importance of choice in the chapter on Empowerment, but it is worth revisiting because here, we encourage the child to vocalize. Let's move beyond forced-choice questions, especially those that can be answered by, for example, pointing, "a banana or an apple? Blueberries or raspberries? Snow White or Cinderella?" Move into open-ended questions requiring some decision-making: "Which book would you like to read tonight? Or "Which winter coat do you want to wear?" or

"Where would you like to go today?" Ask the question and wait for the answer. Aside from encouraging vocalization, choices significantly impact your child's ability to express themselves, grow in confidence, and begin to self-advocate.

Good practice

Avoid labels. When you give a child a label and place them into specific categories, you threaten their self-confidence. Children easily conform to identities given to them by their parents and guardians, making it extremely difficult for them to find their voice and identity. Don't compare them with their siblings or with other children. I remember once asking a boy with ASD why he said something inappropriate. He responded: "It's because of my autism."

Children can grab on to opinions that parents aren't even aware they have communicated. For example, a parent might say a child is the smart one, the intelligent one, or the considerate one. This also applies to negative opinions such as the mean one, the silly one, or the insensitive one. Keep compliments simple, especially in the presence of siblings. If a child has done something funny or clever, instead of saying, "She is the funny one," you could say, "That was very funny." Focusing on the behavior, rather than labeling the child, gives the child room to grow in the case of bad behavior and relieves them of unnecessary pressure in the case of good conduct—model good practice. Keep your eyes open for unexpected moments to model assertiveness and vocalization.

Teaching by example is one of the best ways to demonstrate to your child that it is okay to speak up when necessary. How can you do this? As your child listens, you can tell someone you respect their opinion but see things differently. Later you might process the experience out loud in front of your child, "I felt like I disagreed with her, but I know her opinion has value, so I chose to tell her that." If your child finds these confrontations anxiety-provoking, you can also model that: "I felt nervous about telling her that I disagree, but I told her anyway." You don't need to tell your child they should 'do the same.' Your actions will speak much louder than your words.

You can also share real examples of impactful experiences in your life when you had to speak up and be assertive, especially when you notice that they are trying to do the same thing. Such stories can validate a child who has had the same experience. Finally, you can start your conversation with a statement such as, 'I understand what you are going through because something similar once happened to me."

You can share stories about how you handled the situation and tell them what you would have done differently had you been given a chance to try again. When you do this, they see you as someone who overcame a similar obstacle, assuring them that they can do the same. It also helps them feel like you understand and that they are not alone.

ENCOURAGEMENT

I was speaking to a music teacher recently. She told me a story about a first-grade student with Asperger's syndrome. This student announced in unequivocal terms, "I hate music!" The student became more and more troublesome over the next two years. He used abusive language, became physically aggressive toward his peers, and had frequent meltdowns.

The teacher scheduled some one-to-one time with the student. During those sessions, she discovered that the computer-loving student had learning difficulties. The teacher encouraged him to practice playing some instruments in the staff room and later shared a music composition software program with him. It was not long before the student had composed a song and performed it in front of his peers. His confidence grew, and he became a professional musician in a well-known band.

Children with special needs are as gifted as any other children. They have special abilities but often need extra support to take advantage of the opportunities. As a result, they become frustrated when they're not understood. Sometimes, as a result, they express this frustration via behavior that pushes others away. Generally, this initiates a vicious cycle. Our children should be encouraged to participate in activities they excel in and activities that capitalize on their strengths.

Encouraging independence

As a responsible parent, you want to provide your special child with the best support and opportunities to maximize their potential while avoiding injury. However, depending on the level and nature of your child's needs, you may be overprotective in your zeal to achieve safe, desired outcomes. While that may keep your child in one piece, it is not ideal if you want to build your child's confidence and independence. Remember that your special child is a child first. Their special needs should not define them or unnecessarily hold them back.

Avoid doing everything for your child. Instead, encourage them to brush their teeth and hair and get dressed. Let them help with household chores such as laundry, meal preparation, and clean-up. Of course, some children are not ready or able to engage in certain activities, but remember that you are an expert on your child. You will know if and when your child can step up their participation in household responsibilities. You'll need to step in occasionally, but don't start by instilling doubt in your child.

We have already discussed the importance of choice, which is also relevant here. Let the child choose from a selection of outfits and what to wear. Let them choose which extra-curricular activities to attend and how to get there. If you buy a gadget, let them have a say in the functionalities they would like. If cost is a factor, limit the options to those that suit your budget.

In encouraging independence, don't forget to include some challenging situations that require problem-solving. For example, your child may be about to have dinner, but the table has not been set, or there are no utensils on the table. Some children will wait for the utensils to arrive, and others will ask for them. Encourage them to retrieve the knives and forks for themselves and everyone about to eat. Don't do everything for your special child. Take every opportunity to teach them and treat them like any other child. Too often, parents focus on the child's disability. If your child takes the initiative to, for example, get utensils without your asking or, even better, to get them for the whole family, do *not* let this go unrecognized. Give them specific praise, "Wow, you saw that we needed knives and forks, so you went and got them. Oh, thank you!"

Social skills are essential for lifelong success. Parents must teach their children to develop these skills to encourage independence because children with special needs often struggle in these areas. They may have difficulty greeting others properly or playing with other children. The absence of those skills could translate later into occupational challenges. To build these skills, give your child opportunities to interact with other children. Coach them and invite trustworthy adults to coach them when it is helpful. Your child can hone their social skills during play dates or in extracurricular clubs and groups. It is beneficial if your child can engage with other children in something they enjoy. This helps the child identify their strengths rather than struggle with their weaknesses. Many of our children have cognitive delays and motor deficits that impede them. Unfortunately, these challenges attract bullying, exclusion, and feelings of being isolated. While parents can't make this go away entirely, if they empower their children to the best of their ability, they'll be better able to cope with the circumstances. Keep your eyes open for extracurricular clubs that practice inclusion and teach the children to find and value each other's strengths and work together despite differences and weaknesses.

Role modeling

Families of children with special needs face additional difficulties, but your choice to rise to the challenge with a positive outlook will affect your ability to inspire and empower your child. If you encounter problems head-on with available help, your kids will follow your example and learn to do the same. But, of course, the converse is true; modeling pessimism will breed pessimism.

Model social skills and demonstrate appropriate behavior for your child to see. Be a role model of kindness, patience, and forgiveness. In this way, you will show them what positive relationships look like so that they can also reflect positivity in their lives.

A child must see themselves represented in others. They need to see and learn about great people who became successful despite their disabilities and special needs. Sharing examples will help them begin to see and believe that they, too, can accomplish a lot. Here are a few role models: Temple Grandin, who has autistic spectrum disorder, is an accomplished animal scientist. Steven Speilberg, who has ADHD, is a successful film director. Carol Greider, who has learning disabilities, is a Nobel Prize-winning geneticist. One of our favorites is Helen Keller, who was deaf and blind but became a disability activist and prolific writer.

You and your child will undoubtedly be encouraged by creating a list of people who changed the world despite their special needs and disabilities. Give it a strong title such as: Powerful People with Special Needs and Disabilities Who Changed the World. Don't pressure your child by suggesting they could be on the list. Instead, let them naturally begin to develop their vision for their life.

Encourage learning

Explore apps and other technologies that enhance your child's talents and gifts. There are various apps available with varying functionalities. For example, if your child speaks well but struggles with writing, some apps have a speech-to-text feature that helps them put their words into writing. If they are good at writing but struggle with speech, there are apps with synthesized voices that support communication.

Strength-based learning strategies focus on the individual's strengths, enabling them to identify, articulate, and apply skills relevant to their learning needs. This learner-centred approach requires you to find opportunities for your child to get out and get involved with activities they enjoy. Identify your child's strengths and design strategies that put those abilities to the test. For example, if your child is good at drawing but struggles with reading, let them use their drawing skills to illustrate what they are reading. If your child is a gifted knitter but has trouble with numeracy, you can have them design a piece of fabric with rows and columns that increase by ten. The idea is to find a child's strength and build on it in a way that bypasses or even addresses their weaknesses. Keep some at home if your child is good with visuals and uses them in school. You can also create a system of rewards at home to appreciate a job well done in school. For example, if your child had a successful day, you can take them to the mall for ice cream or another reward.

Be supportive of your child's passion. Provided it's a legitimate option, support your teenagers in their choices and keep it positive. Remember that your children are individuals with unique thoughts, identities, gifts, and talents. They may make choices you don't like, but letting them lead will show them that they are independent people with independent decisions. Also, keep an eye out for opportunities to teach them that with rights come responsibilities.

Their progress might be slow and their accomplishments few, but you must encourage them anyway. Your child must know that you love them unconditionally and support them in whatever they choose.

KEY POINTS OF CHAPTER 5

> Amazing things do not happen overnight. A lot of time and effort will go into seeing your child progress, but it will happen. This is true for most children, especially for differently abled children. Continue to love them and be patient. Control your emotions and manage your frustration; time is a great healer. LISTEN to your child and understand that they're ORIGINAL. They have unique thoughts, opinions, and desires that they can VOCALIZE. Your job is to ENCOURAGE them—to support them and build on their skills and talents. This is the LOVE Game Strategy.

Chapter 6

POTENTIAL:
The PEACE Promotion Formula

In order to move forward, sometimes you've got to stand still
—Andrea Campbell

The PEACE Promotion Formula appreciates the distance travelled and the need for recalibration where necessary. We will cover the subheadings: Practice, Evaluation, Achievement, Creativity and Esteem.

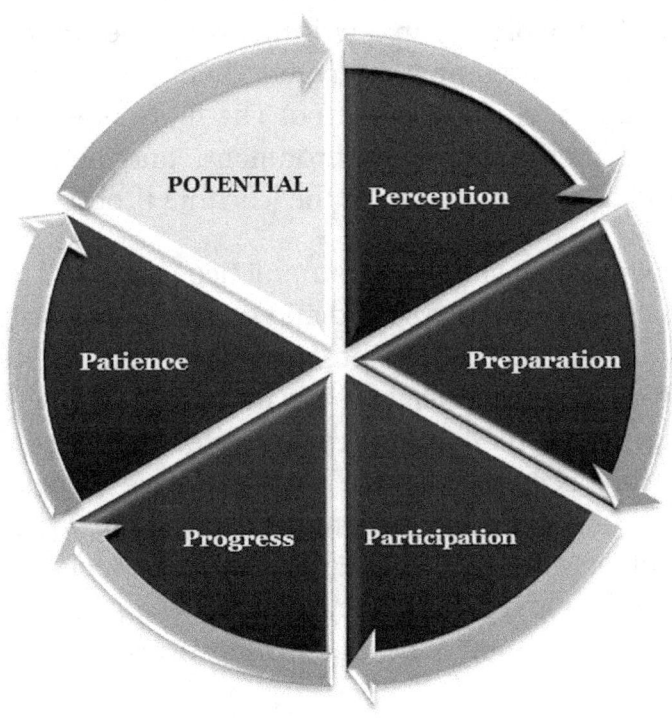

PRACTICE

Parents and educators frequently make mistakes when helping children with special needs. First, they limit their learning to the school environment. Of course, the classroom might be the primary instruction location, but learning should extend to all areas of a child's life.

Think of classroom learning as an initial investment that will yield even higher profits with consistent attention. Take every opportunity to practice the lessons learned. As your child grows, they will find great joy in learning. Don't be afraid to give your child responsibility for their learning. Children take greater ownership of their learning when they have a certain level of control over the experience.

Practice giving your child the opportunity to have direct input into their social and educational choices. Give them options. When working on a writing project, let them choose a topic that inspires and motivates them. Let them choose their extracurricular activities too. The more power you give them over methodology, environment, and activities, the more motivated they will be in the learning process.

Show enthusiasm while you practice with your children. I realize many parents are tired and unable to be enthusiastic in every situation. Do your best when you can. Enthusiasm rubs off on children. They enjoy new activities even more when they notice that adults are interested too. If a child sees that you are keen on helping them practice things they've learned, they will also become enthusiastic. Whether in school subjects or extracurricular activities such as sports, drama, and art, it's necessary to help them practice and share their excitement about their discoveries.

Maximize time and money

There is a plethora of information about time management, but much less on time maximization. Maximizing your time is about prioritizing and doing what is truly important to you. It also includes multitasking, the main difference between time maximizing and time management. When you maximize time, you acknowledge that it is a valuable resource you can't afford to waste. You can, for example, listen to music while driving; or comb your child's hair while watching a television program.

In the same way, you can listen to music while driving, or you can use the time to practice a lesson with your child. You can practice singing, counting, reading number plates, and studying the traffic lights. You can listen to a kid's audiobook that the whole family enjoys.

Teach your child about the places and spaces around them, and if they can, ask them to draw a map of the region or the surrounding businesses such as shops, roads, cars, and parks. If your child is older, you can take this opportunity to teach them the meanings of road signs and road rules. If your child will one day learn to drive, this is an excellent way to start teaching them how to, long before they take the wheel.

Many parents avoid the topic of money management; schools don't generally teach it either. Yet, managing money is a life skill. Be on the lookout for teachable moments when you can engage your kids in meaningful discussions, especially if they understand the concepts. Always be willing to answer their questions and explain your choices. If your child asks for something, take the opportunity to explain the difference between needs, wants, and wishes. If you use a debit or credit card, teach them how both cards work.

Although you teach the child about buying in-store and online, you should be careful not to give the children access to your personal identification number (PIN). This is not because you lack trust in the child; it is a safeguard for you. We have heard many stories where children make in-app purchases that parents have to repay. Limit freedom until you are certain that your child is responsible enough to use a charge card.

Focus on learning

You might be curious what your child scored on their math test when they get home from school. Resist the urge to ask immediately. Why are grades so important? Instead of focusing on their grade, ask them to tell you what they learned in school today. Focus on the child's progress instead of their performance in a particular field. Most parents want their children to achieve highly—to be the best they can be. This aspiration is not bad in and of itself. However, it can become problematic if they put undue pressure on the child and themselves. Remember, they are competing against themselves, not against others. Of course, performance is important, but when you focus on their experiences more than their grades, the child understands that 1) actual learning is more important than grades obtained on a particular test; 2) results are not the main things in life; 3) you value them and their experiences more than their performances; 4) they understand that putting what they've learned into their own words is more important than grades and scores.

Helping your child stay organized is an excellent way to help them feel motivated to learn. Let them organize their learning materials, sports equipment, art materials, etc. Disorganization is a common challenge among most children; it quickly makes them feel overwhelmed and frustrated. Be patient with your child, but be consistent in helping them stay organized in all areas of their lives. As a result, they will feel more in control of their lives and less overwhelmed by the surrounding clutter.

The whole idea behind this practice is to help your child understand that learning isn't limited to the school environment. You can learn at the grocery store, in the backyard, in the car, while watching a movie, and helping in the kitchen. Make the process fun, and be open to learning from your children.

EVALUATION

Build evaluation systems based on your learning goals. Goal setting is an excellent way to build a child's confidence and teach them life skills such as self-awareness, problem-solving, communication, teamwork, and creativity. In addition, it will help the child develop persistence – an essential skill in achieving goals.

The goals and evaluation mechanisms will differ depending on the child's age, abilities, dreams, and strengths. You can set long-term and short-term goals or focus on learning and habits. Children who understand the importance of goal setting are well prepared for successful lifelong learning. Goals may be set based on grades, i.e. academic performance, or on occupational skills such as using cutlery or getting dressed. There are also habit-based goals such as social interaction with peers or reading a story before bed.

Whatever goal you target, make sure it is specific, measurable, attainable, and relevant to the child. This way, you will have a framework to evaluate and measure progress. If it feels like progress is slow or halted, remember that no one moves upwards all the time. We must stop, recalibrate, sometimes step back, and then go again. The key is to build on what you have and keep going as long as possible. Recognise that the very ability to embark and progress on this journey is success in itself. There are minor destinations along the way, and we must never forget to celebrate our small wins.

Goal setting

You should always start with short-term goals that can be met within a few days or weeks. These goals are an excellent way to introduce the child to habitual and educational goals. In addition, short-term goal setting and evaluation will help your child appreciate their progress. As they accomplish these goals, their confidence will grow. Some short-term goals include painting a small picture, completing 100 jumps on the trampoline, and learning ten new words.

With a long-term goal, your child focuses on an ongoing project and works toward completion. Your child may need more help with these goals and may need to draw from varying sources. Help them with their long-term goals. This will teach them the concept of continuous focus and determination and how smaller efforts add up to more significant achievements. In addition, this will help them learn to plan, think about what lies ahead, and understand that some things in life take time.

Long-term goals teach children patience, motivation, growth, achievement of short-term goals, and hard work. Make sure your child understands that things might not always progress as planned, but this should not hinder us from continuing to work towards our goals. Some children need extra encouragement to achieve their goals, whereas others need additional time to get to the same point as others. Sometimes the plans change altogether. It's okay for your child to change their mind and move in a different direction.

The ultimate goal is for your child to achieve consistent progress in learning and developing skills that position them to take their place in society. Add flexibility to your goals, ensuring you tailor your goals and evaluation methods to your child. Revisit and readjust the goals when necessary, considering any additional resources and support your child may need to achieve them. Consider too if goals need to be simplified and broken into bite-size chunks to have a higher success rate. For example, instead of saying Sue will be able to dress herself by the end of next month, say Sue will be able to put on her shoes properly by the end of the month. If Sue can identify the correct shoe for each foot, you may want to include tying her laces. Many of our children have gross and fine motor issues and struggle to tie laces, buckle shoes and button shirts. By adding extra steps, you can build skills in these micro day-to-day tasks that will serve your children for the long haul.

You can work toward reinforced learning and extra tutoring hours or spend more time on homework. Children who attend special schools often have practical assignments such as stringing beads or dressing a doll. These activities help their motor skills, communication skills and teamwork ability. Maybe your child's schedule or learning tools need reorganization. For example, some children may benefit from having a visual board with a written list and pictures of the steps you need to follow to achieve a particular goal. You should choose an approach that works for you and your child and helps them keep track of their academic, social, and occupational goals.

Consolidation

Once your child has achieved a goal, give them plenty of opportunities to practice. For example, don't be tempted to continue to dress your child if they have learned to do this themselves. Instead, start working on other skills or increase the difficulty level. Encourage your child to try new skills. Encourage and praise their efforts and build on a foundation of love.

Every time a goal is achieved, celebrate with your child. I am in parent forums often, and it is incredible to see the feats parents celebrate. The online community of parents of children with special needs is very supportive and candid in talking about their children managing to "do a poo" or being finally able to take a step at the age of four. These joys would be lost on most parents of neurotypical children. This camaraderie validates the need to connect with parents of children with similar diagnoses. They understand your journey and can support and encourage you when you need it most.

Celebrations don't have to be a big deal. They include intangible rewards such as a high-five, a trip to the local mall, or a picnic in the park. They also include morale-boosting acts such as a one-minute ceremony to hang a child's painting in a prominent spot, along with applause by the family. Tangible gifts of toys, gadgets and other items that appeal to the child are also in order.

Encouragement, praise, and positive affirmations boost your child's self-confidence and help them stay motivated and committed to achieving their goals. Goal setting and evaluating those goals will help your child stay on track in school and at home. Know the types of goals to set, how best to evaluate them, and when you've achieved them. Consistent actions in this regard will build character and success for you and your child.

Achievement

Your child's self-esteem gets a boost when you reward their small, everyday wins. Your child's achievement directly correlates with your level of encouragement and support. We all love the significant gains, but we must never forget the tiny wins that lead to them. Your child may not yet be able to dress himself, but the fact that he can put on his Velcro shoes is a big achievement worth honouring.

Graduation can be an exciting time! For most teens, it represents caps and gowns, diplomas, and summer internships followed by job hunting and the start of careers. It can also mean getting ready to attend the college or university of their choice. The season is bittersweet because parents and children are excited to close one chapter of their lives and open the next, but they're unsure of what lies ahead. Many parents feel the future holds a lot of promise for their children. This is a time of transition that signifies growth from childhood to adulthood and the heady mix of freedom and responsibility both bring.

However, for parents of children with special needs, the thought of graduation looming may cause fear, anxiety, and uncertainty instead of excitement and hope. One way of minimizing these emotions is to remember that your child is unique. My little girl will graduate in her way. Ceaseless exams and demands will not pressure her—she is running in her own lane. I understand that most of us would prefer if our special child were not so special, that she fit in with the crowd. However, you must remember and accept that your child stands out at this point in your life. Celebrate the difference. Take time to reflect on everything your child has achieved thus far. Celebrate the transition to adulthood or to the next phase in their life, and be grateful for how far you've come.

Transition planning

Create a transition plan for the next step of your child's life, considering their strengths, interests, talents, abilities, and gifts. Document their needs and state how they will be met in the short, medium, and long terms. Assess your child's skills and make plans to fill any gaps. Review and revise their education plan to ensure enough progression routes are built into the current plan. Create a thorough, well-rounded plan by gathering and including input from therapists, doctors, teachers, siblings, support staff, friends, and other people in your child's life. Every plan will be different, but it should generally cover independent living, community involvement, further education, employment, and social interaction.

Different school districts have diverse policies, but it is customary to create a transition strategy when your child is thirteen and in their later teens. These policies may vary, but your educational institution can guide you. In this plan, your child's interests and goals are analyzed, and different parties are identified regarding their role in implementation.

If your child can pursue higher education, options include vocational training, university, and technical education. If your child enrols into any of these institutions, ascertain the available services early on and inform them of your child's special needs in writing. Your child has the same educational rights as any other student in the education system. This means that your child's institution of choice must make the necessary adjustments to give your child an equal opportunity to participate in all programs with reasonable adjustments made.

Employment

Your child has desires and aspirations like everyone else. Do not assume they don't want to pursue a career because they have special needs. If they can work, you must support and empower them. Consider the jobs and relevant activities that suit their skills, abilities, and interests. Look for ways to use their strengths to be productive and support themselves. For example, if your child is an animal lover and knows how to relate to animals, they might aim for a job in a local pet shop or as a veterinarian.

In their teenage years, your child can do volunteer or paid work to see if their interests turn into long-term employment opportunities. Many schools work with vocational educational institutions and training organizations to arrange apprenticeships, traineeships, internships, and work experiences.

Independent living

Young adults with special needs can live independently, in group homes, or supported accommodation if they require full-time help. Your strategy should include their plans and goals, but it should also consider a realistic assessment of their skills and the need to be safe while living independently. The skills should include self-care skills and life skills such as time management, handling finances, doing their laundry, shopping, cleaning, cooking, and transportation.

Your strategy must include relevant ideas to keep friendships intact, meet and interact with new people, and participate in social and community events. Your child might also be interested in recreational, social, and community activities they enjoy, such as exercise classes and going to the movies. They may also want to try something new. It's good to look into available services for children and young adults with special needs in your local area. You may find services that help with routine activities such as grocery shopping, group social outings, movies with others, and working out in nature or a gym.

Reviewing the strategy

Your child might change their mind. They might also learn skills at a different pace than you expect. For these reasons, it is imperative to review the plan regularly. This review can be once or twice a year or a few months before or after the transition. It's important to involve teachers and other professionals in the review process, and you always want to involve your child and ask them how to move forward. Talking with your child is the best way to understand their thoughts, if their plans have changed, and if they need help.

CREATIVITY

There isn't a one-size-fits-all way to teach a child. Learning is a process, and it can happen anywhere and with anything. It's incumbent upon the parents to strive toward supporting all the dimensions of their children's well-being. This includes cognitive growth, mental, social and emotional health, character development, and interpersonal skills. Your child's creativity is a vital part of what makes them unique. When we help our children to develop creativity, they build resolve, inquiry, independence, positivity, confidence, ingenuity, problem-solving and coping skills. It is therefore important to nurture creativity.

A well-rounded education focuses on academics and non-academic teaching and learning activities. Creating an environment where a child can explore his creative potential is a necessary complement to that package of intervention. Use innovative strategies to hold your child's attention and keep them interested in learning. Teaching shouldn't be limited to formal lessons, worksheets, and tests. Some of the best educational opportunities occur when children are completely unaware of them. Undoubtedly you have already begun to develop an arsenal of ideas to exercise creativity. Below are some ideas on the matter:

Learners and aspects of creativity

There is no reason why a visually impaired child cannot be encouraged to write a poem. A child with dyslexia can compose a beautiful melody, and a child with autism can inspire an invention or create a striking collage. A high-functioning student can draw an insightful and intricate design. Each learner is being stretched differently by engaging the mind and tapping into their creativity. They must be encouraged to do so, even if it's a monumental effort. As parents, you must be there to help your child make the right choices for creativity. Help them step outside of comfort zones, try new approaches, test limits, and explore new perspectives. This can be difficult for some children depending on their level of ability. Some children may be challenged to start an activity, while others might struggle to sustain momentum and keep going to the end. This can also be said of the general population, so your kids are not all that different. Even the most advanced learners have trouble engaging and persisting with creativity. Our children may need extra encouragement, assistance, reinforcement, or guidance to tap into and maximize their strengths, talents, interests, energy, effort, and coping mechanisms.

Nurturing creativity

Nurturing creativity is not a top-down process—it is a collaborative one, with the child taking the lead where possible. Here are a few suggestions for parents, caregivers, and teachers of learners with special needs.

Labeling - You can label objects around the house such as doors, windows, chairs, kitchen, plants, bathroom, and items on a bookshelf. Write the words in bold and use colored paper or colored ink to capture and keep their attention. Soon your child will associate words with objects, and you'll both have fun in the process.

Exploring stars - Nights are magical, especially when the sky is full of stars. A beautiful sky is an excellent playground for a child's imagination and curious nature. You can take that opportunity to help the child see the beauty of the world, and both of you can research and talk about planets, constellations, galaxies, and shooting stars. At the elementary level, ask your child to count the stars.

Outdoor exploration - Nature has a lot to offer; the choices are inexhaustible. Watch the clouds on a sunny or rainy day. Name the different types of clouds and ask your child what they think of them. What shapes and colors can they see? What creatures can they spot in the clouds? On a rainy day, can they see a rainbow? Take a sketchbook and draw the clouds. If your child is so inclined, you can complete additional research on clouds and take the discussion further. Picking flowers is another outdoor activity that can foster creativity. Let your child name the colours, compile bunches into a bouquet, or braid the grass blades.

Shopping classes - Trips to the store can be overwhelming for our children. It takes some time to understand that they are not permitted to pick the items from the shelves and eat them in the store. Once you manage those dynamics, you can take advantage of your shopping trips by turning them into teaching experiences. Include your child in the shopping tasks, enlist their help writing a list, and select items. You can discuss the best way to find affordable items at each store and let them point out any discounted items. Take the opportunity to teach them about money—let them occasionally pay the cashier. Remember, these lessons will go a long way when they live independently.

Creative cooking - Cooking is a fun experience for children, and there are myriad opportunities to learn new concepts. Include them in mixing, whisking, stirring, beating, peeling, tasting and the range of other activities in the kitchen. You can make cooking a joyful educational experience by talking about what you are doing and the implements you use in the process. You can encourage your child to read recipes or name the ingredients. You can also challenge them to practice math skills by measuring ingredients. Adding yeast to the dough and watching it rise is a real-life chemistry experiment you both can enjoy. If unsure how it works, research the process and explain it to your child. If the child is willing and able, you can let them plan and prepare a healthy, economical meal under your supervision. It may be messy at first, so be prepared to help clean up. It's a small price to pay, considering that you are empowering them to develop independence for the future.

Strategies for crafting a creative environment

Help your child develop a strong appreciation for creativity. This will help them build intelligence and achieve success and fulfilment. Here are other factors to consider.

Support networks - Help your child tap into support networks. Friends, family members, caregivers, teachers, and others can offer support. Children who perceive the adults in their lives as being caring, respectful, willing, and available to help are more motivated to exercise their creativity.

Imagination - Consider what will inspire children and spark their imagination. Language stimulation, sensory experiences, and ample opportunities for unstructured play and discovery can stimulate creativity alone and with others. In addition, your child can benefit from exploring music, art, puzzles, dance, exercise, and discovery walks. The use of assistive technology may also be beneficial.

The need for balance - Ensure children have a healthy mix of learning opportunities, physical exercise, social activities, sleep, and family time. Also, encourage time for tranquillity—meditation and solitude, quiet time for innovation and exploration. All of these experiences can stimulate creativity.

Self-belief - Encourage your child to have faith in their abilities. When initial attempts fail, kids can experience frustration and doubt their capability. Help your child realize and accept their limitations but build their self-belief in their strengths. Help them learn that failure is a step on the path to success and, when they succeed, celebrate with them. Remember that although creativity may seem complicated, it can be a means of bypassing a roadblock.

Positivity - A positive outlook and a can-do mindset empower and bolster self-confidence. Celebrating the small steps and accomplishments creates an environment where optimism, positivity and creativity can thrive. Don't focus on what didn't work; keep an open mind and maintain a positive attitude.

Goals - It helps to ensure that IEP goals are aligned effectively with the child's needs. When an educational program is appropriate, such that a child progresses and feels positive about learning, it sets the stage for inquiry, a sense of purpose, meaningful connections, and creative expression.

ESTEEM

At a time when children are exposed to social media, fake news, online bullies, and rapidly changing social expectations, it can be tough to make sure they grow up with a positive self-image. But, as parents, we are responsible for putting time and energy into helping our children develop positive self-esteem to become happy, secure adults.

Children with a learning disability are often the brunt of jokes, and they suffer more bullying than their neurotypical peers. You must keep a keen eye on this—especially if your child is non-verbal. Sometimes you can ask for feedback from parents of other children in your child's class or teachers. This may help you to discern whether it is a battle your child can manage on their own or one that needs support. If you are concerned about what you hear, speak to the school about your concerns.

Because children with special needs face a broad spectrum of emotional, behavioral and educational challenges, developing self-esteem is not as straightforward as it might be for a neurotypical child. It's not always easy for parents and caregivers to talk to their children about intimacy and relationships, but as they grow, our children experience the same feelings, risks and environmental factors as neurotypical kids. Children with disability are at a higher risk of abuse and neglect, so parents must do all they can to help them navigate their feelings and sustain healthy relationships. Empower them to stay safe while building their self-esteem and life chances.

Positive self-esteem remains essential for general well-being. Creating an environment where a child feels accepted, loved, and safe gives rise to self-esteem development. Notwithstanding any anxieties you may experience, the kids need to know that they are accepted, celebrated and loved for who they are. This means recognizing their unique limits and abilities even as you support your child's progress in these areas.

Esteem building strategies

Watching your child struggle to complete a task can be heartbreaking for parents. As a parent, you often want to alleviate any pain your child experiences. Unfortunately, this is not always possible or helpful for your child. Let's look at strategies to help your child develop a positive self-image and become strong, resilient, and self-confident. These strategies will help them face their challenges with greater strength.

Make them feel special - Show your child you value him just as he is. Set aside time to spend with your child each week—when they can anticipate having your undivided attention and enjoying each other's company by doing an activity of the child's choosing. I take my daughter to the local park, where we go for a walk and watch the birds on the lake.

Capitalize on strengths - Make a list of all the activities your child excels in and post it in a prominent place in the home. Use both words and pictures and draw attention to them often. Talk to your child about their strengths and constantly remind them of their abilities. For example, I tell my child daily that she is beautiful and clever.

Embrace problem-solving - Good problem-solving abilities are a confidence booster. Help your child develop coping strategies for dealing with daily struggles and dilemmas. Avoid the temptation of rushing in with your solutions. Instead, encourage your child to think outside of the box. If they get stumped, offer choices and help them find workable solutions. Always remember to encourage and reassure them. Earlier, I mentioned my daughter and I singing, "I can do it." When we sing that song, it inspires her to try harder. Find a strategy that works for you.

Responsibilities and opportunities - Self-esteem increases when children contribute to other people's well-being. Let them feel useful—send them on errands or ask them to put on their shoes, for example. This participation conveys the message that they are able and have something of value to offer. Give your child responsibility for tasks and projects and let them have the freedom to make decisions. Responsibilities and decisions help them own their power and build their self-esteem.

This decision-making might seem insignificant to you because you make thousands of decisions every day, but the decision-making power of many children is minimal. When you trust them with something simple and acknowledge when they do it correctly, their self-confidence grows significantly. Where possible and appropriate, find ways for your child to volunteer in the community. Frequent positive steps are the building blocks to greater improvement in self-worth and self-confidence.

Create leadership opportunities - Create games where the child is responsible for allocating tasks to participants. When doing academic work at home, allow your child to lead the sequence or determine start and finish times. Those are ways to tailor your intervention and help your child learn to take decisions.

You may be able to find organizations in your vicinity that provide leadership programs that your child can access. When you inquire about these programmes, let the organizers know about your child's diagnosis. Then, to avoid disappointment, find out if their programs will be a good fit for your child before signing up.

Be realistic - Be truthful to yourself about what you can expect your child to accomplish in a given task. This does not mean you put limits on your child; it means you are realistic and accept the child as he is. Children take their emotional cues from the adults around them. So if you are fussed about a situation, they will be too. Misconceptions can be a source of pain for children, but realistic expectations help them develop a sense of control—a key ingredient in esteem building.

Tangible rewards - Gifts and rewards are always welcome boosts. One such reward is a success jar which is an excellent way to remind your child of past victories from the smallest to the biggest. Success jars are very easy to make. You need a large, clear plastic container and some slips of paper. Sit with the child from time to time and ask them about everything they've done well. For children who are non-verbal, you will need to be creative. Use pictures and words. The blank cards supplied with the Pocket Learner are beneficial. Prompt the children when necessary and show enthusiasm as you select the cards. Place the slips in the container and read them out to the child when they are having a bad day or feeling discouraged. Remind them how it felt when they first achieved whatever is written on the paper, and tell them they are still the same person who was great that day. Keep adding to your lists.

Sports - Participating in sports is an effective confidence-builder in children. The sport can be a team or solo game and should match their abilities, age, talents, and interests. Once you identify a sport your child enjoys, focus on it and find someone who can help them build on their natural ability. Sports teach children perseverance, teamwork, hard work, training, discipline, commitment, the feel-good attitude of working toward a group goal, and the joy of sharing this passion with others. Like many other hobbies, sports can give a child a strong sense of identity, which is crucial in building self-esteem.

Positive self-talk - Nurturing positive self-talk in children with special needs is probably the most important factor in this list. Teach your child that nobody is perfect, even you as a parent. Help them understand that we all have intrinsic value even with our imperfections, and we are unique. We must all be proud of ourselves. Teach your child a growth mindset, and encourage them to go for what they want because they can achieve anything they put their minds to. Start using positive words such as "excited" instead of "nervous" or "challenging" instead of "impossible." Most importantly, teach by example. Teach your child to see the lesson and opportunity in failure. Help them know the importance of affirmations and positive self-talk from within. Positive self-talk nurtured consistently can be a powerful tool in teaching children self-confidence and self-worth.

KEY POINTS OF CHAPTER 6

> Children enjoy friendships, and they love to play. Use these natural interests and outlets to teach them new skills and help them PRACTICE what they have learned. Use play and other creative ways to help them learn physical, social, emotional, and communication skills. Set short and long-term goals for your child to achieve, then EVALUATE those goals to understand your child's progress. Reflect on your ACHIEVEMENT to date, and develop a plan for things yet to be done. Address challenges with CREATIVITY and increase resilience by building self-ESTEEM. Adjust the goals as necessary, and change course when you need to. You are well on your way to a more sustainable journey in supporting your special child when you apply the PEACE Promotion Formula.

Chapter 7

The Pocket Learner

The parent makes the child and the child makes the parent
—Andrea Campbell

This chapter introduces the Pocket Learner—a tool uniquely developed to empower families to support the learning of children with learning difficulties and those diagnosed with special educational needs and disabilities.

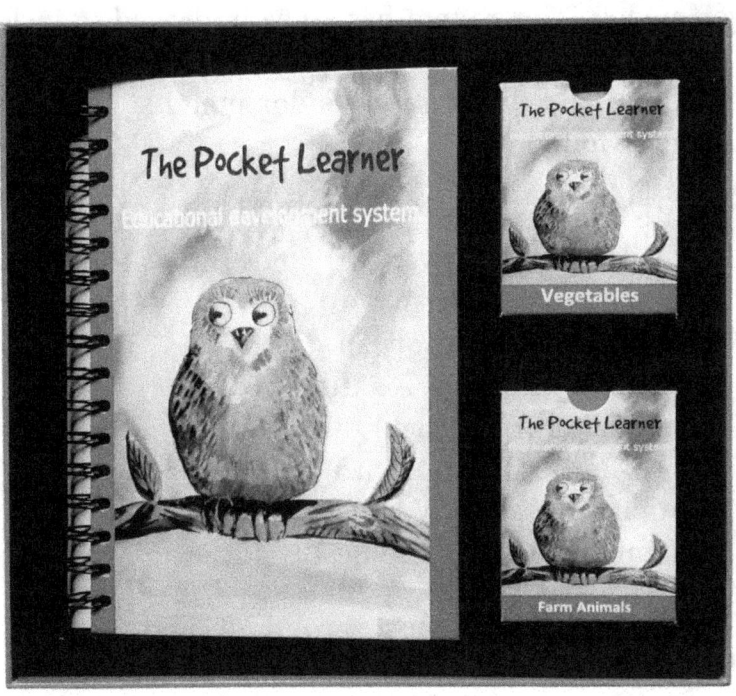

ORIGINS

The Pocket Learner is a multi-award-winning innovative concept which I developed to address the educational needs of my daughter, who had learning difficulties. I believed that my child could achieve more than she was accomplishing in her mainstream school. My frustrations with mainstream education's limited ability to support my daughter and my observations of other families in similar situations gave birth to the development of the Pocket Learner. I realized this system could benefit other families whose children had similar struggles.

The Pocket Learner's journey commenced when I received the first award at the British Invention Show. I took the rudimentary prototype to the show in 2014 and received a silver medal. The system has since improved to include a wide array of resources for which I received several international and innovation endorsements and awards, including the following:

- British Invention Society World Invention Award
- British Female Inventors and Innovators Network International Awards
- International European Women Inventors & Innovators Network Award
- Black Enterprise Mogul Award
- Powerhouse Global Award
- National Business Women's Award
- Chamber of Commerce Best Innovation Award (2x)

The accolade I am most proud of is the medal my daughter brought home – The Jack Petchey Achievement Award for Outstanding Achievers – a national honour she received through her school in 2020.

WHAT IT IS

The Pocket Learner is an educational system that families, teachers, language professionals, speech therapists, special educational needs coordinators, health workers and caregivers use to help children build vocabulary, read, and count. The system uses images, written words, and rewards. It is beneficial in teaching children with special educational needs and disabilities or those experiencing learning difficulties. Although the primary focus is on children with learning disabilities, it is also being used increasingly by education practitioners and those supporting the education of neuro-typical children in their early years in mainstream educational institutions to aid learning, improve communication and develop confidence and self-esteem.

The user-friendly system can be used alongside traditional teaching methodologies, easily fitting into nursery and primary school settings. Users can adapt the training according to the needs of the respective children. The resources include blank cards, which facilitators are encouraged to tailor according to a child's needs. These are particularly useful to parents who wish to complement the learning delivered in mainstream education using traditional teaching methodologies. The materials allow children to progress at their own pace as the system adapts to their different learning styles and needs. It is, however, advisable to have reasonable targets to measure progress.

Children likely to benefit from this program include those with dyslexia, Down's syndrome, developmental delays, speech impediments, hearing issues, and those on the autism spectrum and others. It is built with sturdy materials suitable for multiple uses and consists of a workbook and cards from an ever-expanding range of themes. It is important to note that children who are non-verbal can also use the Pocket Learner. However, it will be most effective for non-verbal learners who can communicate via signs, whether formal sign language or their unique methods of communication. While the Pocket Learner aids speech development, it is primarily a reading and communication tool resource that equips adults working with children struggling in their early years. It provides a fun way for children to learn and boosts their chances to aspire higher and build a foundation that will enable them to serve their unique gifts to the world.

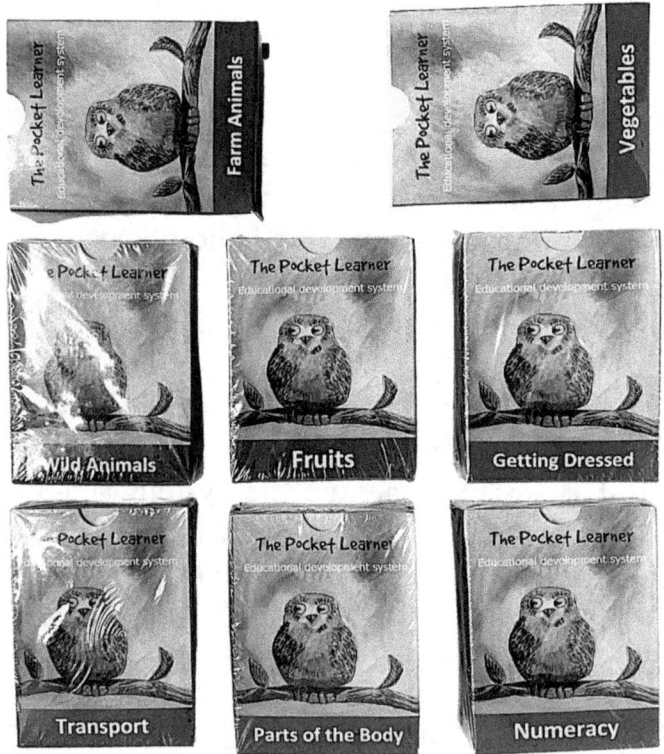

The Pocket Learner's ever-expanding themes

How It Works

The Pocket Learner enables parents and teachers to design and implement a comprehensive and complementary learning programme that can be used consistently to enhance a child's education. It fits in with several bodies of research, and the system has the endorsements of educational professionals, practitioners and parents who have used it successfully.

There are three primary elements of the Pocket Learner—cards with words, cards with pictures, and rewards. The cards are slipped in and out of pockets accompanied by teaching and repetition, association and rewards. The system encourages parents to spark curiosity and invite verbal responses by using the questioning method with their children. This questioning increases the child's use and understanding of language in an engaging and enjoyable way. In time, your child will endeavour to use language spontaneously, particularly when motivated by the rewards.

The Pocket Learner is a holistic educational tool for children with a disability which fits effectively into the Special Education Blueprint. The following is the Pocket Learner methodology for enhanced learning of children with special needs. In essence, the facilitator is directed to:

1) Take leadership of your child's education, development and growth.

2) Promote expression using appropriate methods—speech, signs or body language.

3) Introduce audiovisuals - physical and electronic.

4) Use repetition and reiteration to consolidate learning

5) Provide a nurturing environment for your child to achieve.

6) Actively encourage your child to push themselves and to aim high.

7) Reflect on distance travelled, review, readjust, and redesign support.

The above steps form the acronym: LEARNER, which represents Leadership, Expression, Audiovisuals, Repetition, Nurturing, Encouragement and Reflection. I hope you will use the acronym as a guide when you use the Pocket Learner resources to support your child's educational development.

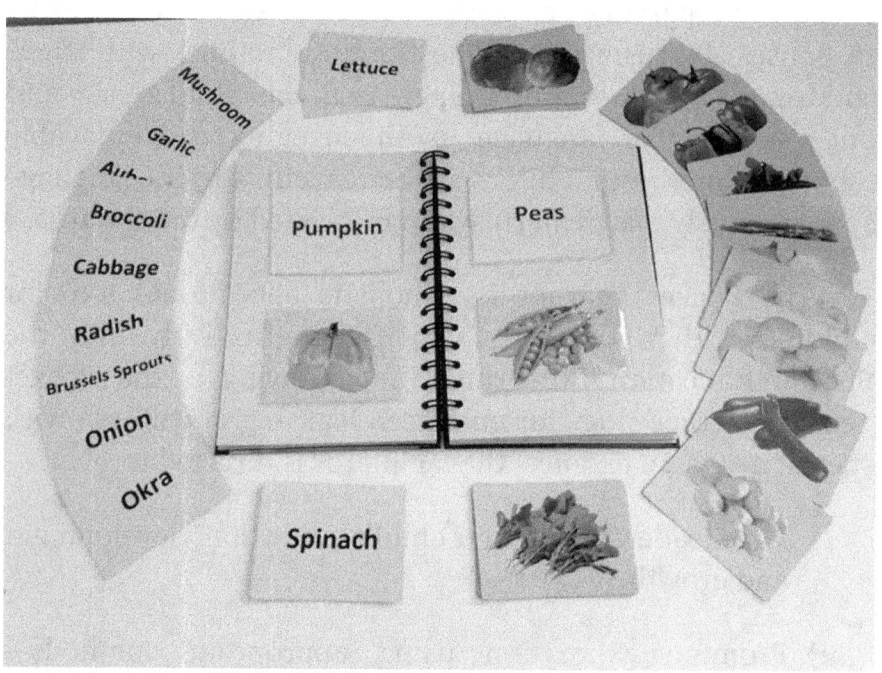

Vocabulary development

Manipulation of the pockets, and a little innovation on your part using cards specifically designed to familiarize your child with the essential words needed at age three and beyond, will ultimately unlock the door to simple but effective communication. Then, your child can start practicing in a familiar, interesting, stimulating, and fun environment. Formal vocabulary building is usually not viewed as a "fun" task and is typically neglected, but with the Pocket Learner, parents and children find learning words enjoyable.

The beauty of the Pocket Learner is that children can learn at their own pace, although it is advisable to set reasonable targets to measure progress. As your child progresses and becomes more relaxed and comfortable with a particular learning style, do not be afraid to engage their imagination with more challenging words. Be proactive and try to encourage the child using a reward structure. Each child has a different currency that gets them excited about progressing. Try varying rewards such as praise, music, or playing with a favourite toy until you discover what best motivates your child. You will need to exercise patience as research studies have shown that in most cases, children should be exposed to words 5-7 times before the words are committed to their long-term memory.

Learning to read

Reading can prove challenging to some as the brain must perform several functions simultaneously to make sense of the written word. Those who find reading difficult may struggle directly or indirectly in life.

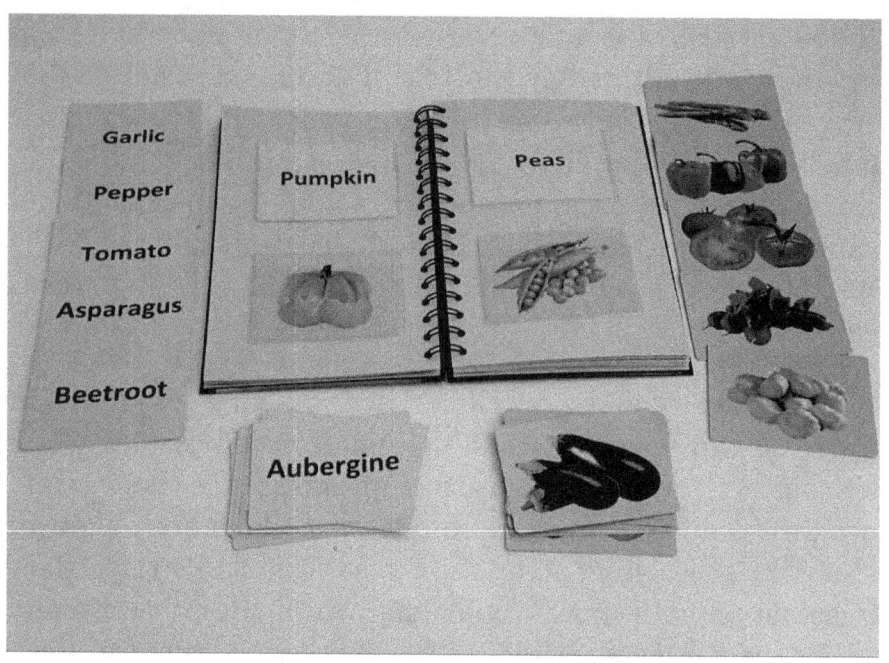

Using the Pocket Learner, your child will learn the names of images and match them to written words. After this, they will learn to identify these words without the pictures and develop their reading skills. The physical resources pair with tangible and intangible rewards that help keep focus. Examples of rewards are praise, clapping, music, treats, toys and hugs. Try different rewards until you discover what best motivates the child.

The Pocket Learner system encourages you to use questioning and encourage curiosity in your child, thus increasing their use and understanding of language. In time your child will endeavour to use language spontaneously, particularly when they crave the rewards you are offering.

Encourage the child to make requests and continuously stretch the vocabulary. For example, give your child an orange and wait for them to ask for help. Teach them to say, "peel it, please", and wait for them to use language. Children with special needs may take longer to respond, so you have to be patient. The Pocket Learner logo—an owl is a poignant reminder of this. The acronym OWL means: Observe, Wait, Listen, bearing in mind that listening is not only to voices but also to body language and other reactions.

The Pocket Learner is a valuable intervention tool for word building, sentence construction, and guided or independent learning. It serves as an ideal platform for developing reading skills. Children use techniques including phonics, repetition, association, reiteration and rewards and generally exhibit great enthusiasm provided the environment is a stimulating one.

Learning to count

Pocket Learner has incorporated a simple but straightforward system for the child to understand the basic foundation of addition, subtraction, multiplication and division. It caters to all four learning styles. Visual learners benefit from the physical resources, auditory learners from the spoken instructions, reading learners can engage with the written words and symbols, and kinesthetic learners can handle the materials and move counters around to solve various mathematical problems.

Adults with at least basic numeracy skills earn approximately 25% more than those without the skills needed to solve elementary mathematical problems. Moreover, when young learners grasp the fundamentals, they are on their way to being numerate and functional in society.

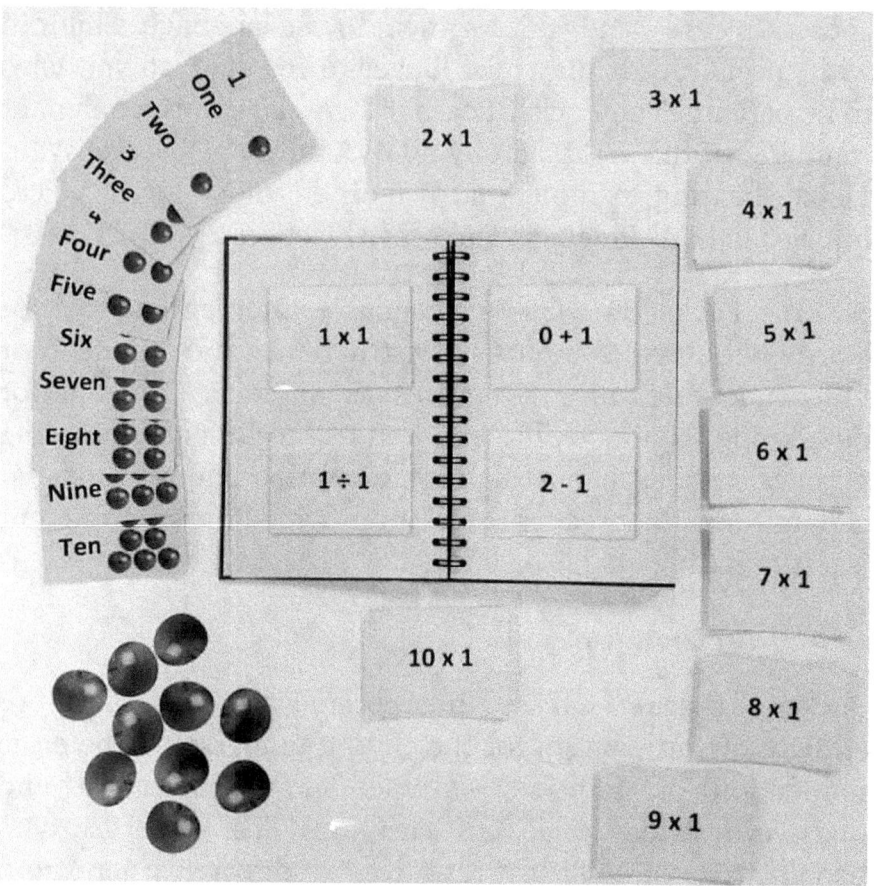

Assessment and revision

The Pocket Learner is ideally suited to support all the fundamentals surrounding assessment and revision by creatively using the pockets to assimilate and digest information.

It is easy to measure progress using the Pocket Learner. A child who previously used only pictures to communicate or who had to point at what they wanted can look at a written word and be able to read or sign it, for example: selecting the word "Milk" to request a glass of milk or "Toilet" to indicate the need to go to the restroom. Encourage the child to practise the words they have learnt. It is both a joyous and a decisive moment and can be a serious game-changer in the lives of all those involved in the child's life when they learn to articulate their needs in this way.

Take some time to review performance and recognise what works well and needs improvement. Then, identify and document the lessons you have learned about yourself and your child, focusing mainly on how you can enhance your performance to support their education.

Rework your strategy to make it more effective in subsequent rounds of support. Be creative in your approach and endeavour to expand your work into other areas such as numeracy and higher education. Consistent use of the program leads to increased and rapid learning, raised aspirations, and greater confidence.

Learning new languages

Learning a new language is a worthwhile endeavor and increases confidence. Holidays to foreign countries become more fun, and less anxiety-provoking; shopping, sightseeing and eating out are less stressful. Also, if you have a good knowledge of the language, you can have meaningful conversations with people you meet. The Pocket Learner enhances vocabulary building and sentence construction in any language you desire, working individually or in a group setting.

Complementary uses

In addition to the above core uses, the Pocket Learner inspires and empowers. It is designed by parents for parents and is effective in building self-esteem and confidence, boosting general knowledge, raising aspirations and ultimately improving a child's opportunities and quality of life.

The system is also used in speech and language therapy to restore speech where illness adversely affects individuals' speech capability. As added benefits, the Pocket Learner stimulates family bonding and promotes inclusion and community cohesion. The act of slotting cards into pockets also stimulates fine motor skills development.

The Pocket Learner additional materials (which are yet to be released) include scheduling cards, nursery and primary table-top and floor resources, card games and charts. Those resources build higher-level skills such as decision-making, problem-solving, negotiation, leadership and emotional intelligence.

THE POCKET LEARNER – KEY RESOURCE IN THE TOOLKIT

The Pocket Learner is the recommended and principal resource in the Special Education Advancement Toolkit. The system enables parents, caregivers and educators to design and implement a comprehensive and complementary learning programme that can be used consistently to enhance their children's education. It fits in with several bodies of research and is a worthy addition to other therapies and educational systems geared at learning development. The unique selling proposition of the Pocket Learner is its flexibility and durability, allowing parents and others using the system to be creative and to widen and deepen the learning goals and outcomes. It complements traditional methodologies employed in mainstream and special education as parents can tailor the cards and acquire new theme cards as their children grow and expand their knowledge.

The Pocket Learner

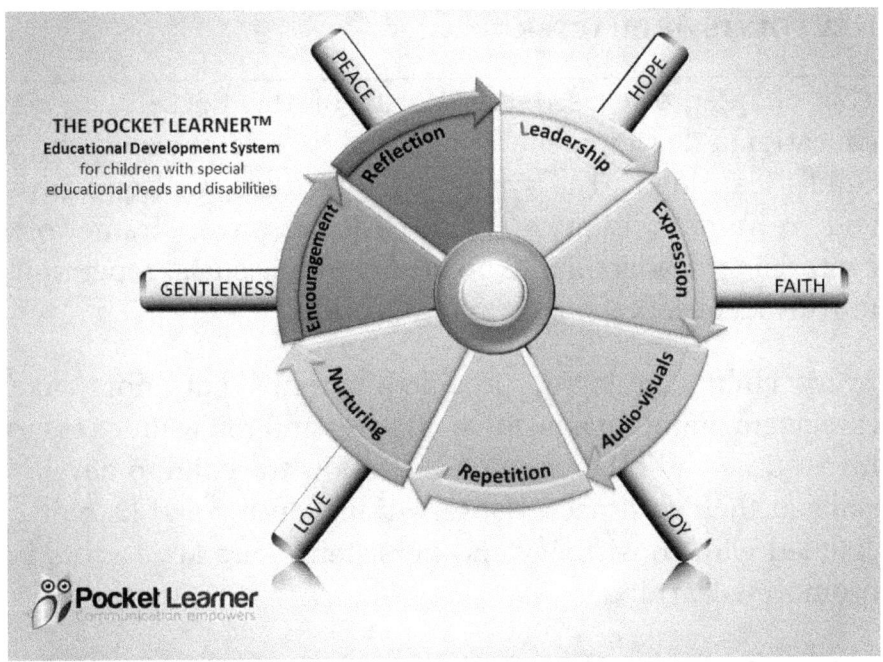

The Pocket Learner fits into the Special Education Advancement Toolkit

Rather than the actual materials, the Pocket Learner's magic is in the learning system. For this reason, the Pocket Learner Educational Development System is a multi-award-winning invention and innovation recognised as a key resource in teaching and learning children and adults with special educational needs and disabilities. For more information, please visit www.pocketlearner.net.

KEY POINTS OF CHAPTER 7

This chapter discussed the merits of the Pocket Learner educational development system and its role in improving a child's learning. The system uses pictures, written words and rewards within a LEARNER acronym framework comprising: leadership, expression, audiovisuals, repetition, nurturing, encouragement and reflection.

Every child can learn, provided parents, educators, and caregivers maintain a positive mindset and the willingness to invest time and other resources to allow the child to develop skills at their own pace. Observation, waiting and listening, coupled with consistency and persistence, are key factors in promoting learning.

The Pocket Learner fits effectively into the Special Education Advancement Toolkit to provide holistic support for children with learning difficulties. When a learning culture is established, practiced and nurtured, success becomes not only attainable but also inevitable.

Conclusion

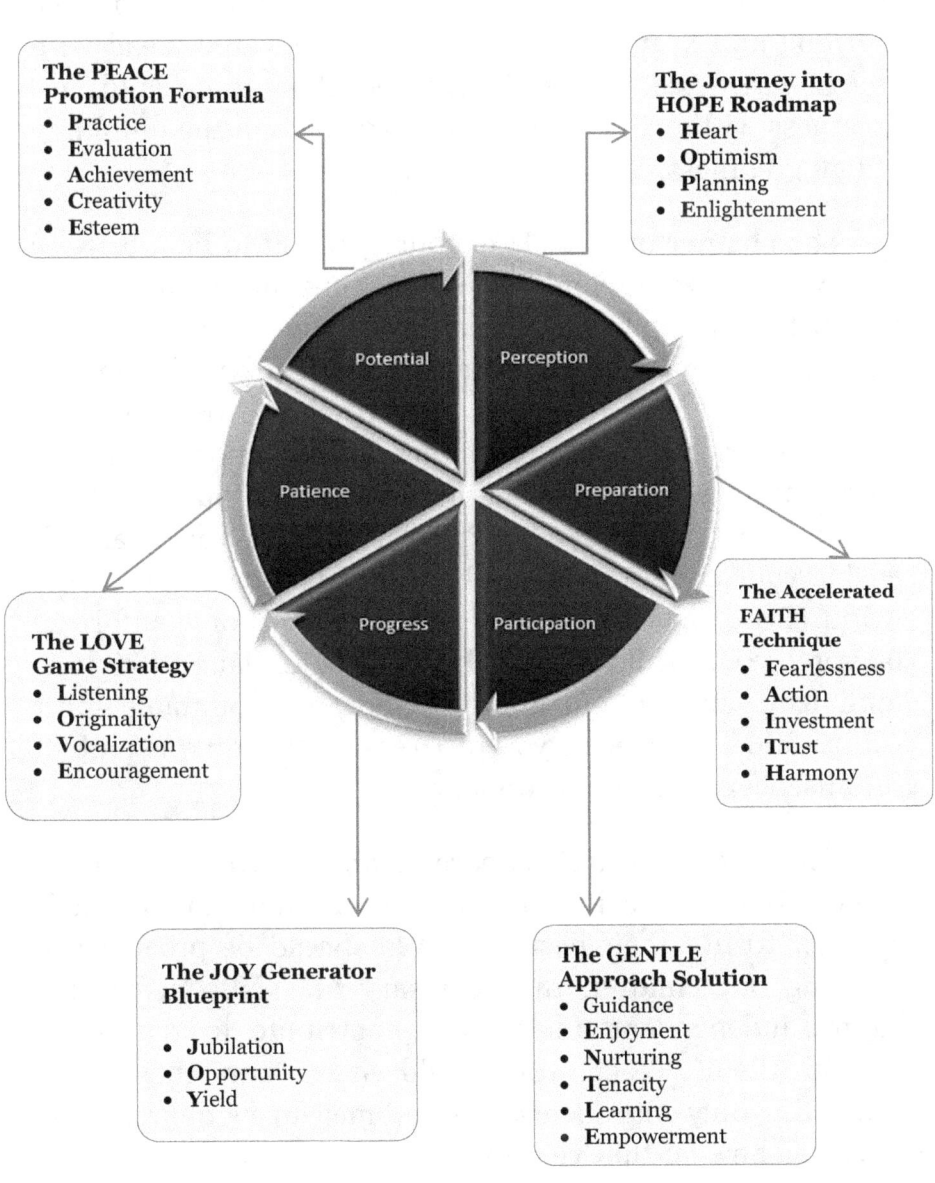

We started our journey with HOPE—a deep desire and expectation for positive change. Build your foundation on hope and optimism, recognizing that your child is a treasure and you have been chosen to grow this treasure. Hope for the future is what gets you out of bed in the morning and keeps you inspired and motivated. Lead with your heart, safe in the knowledge that your child has greatness within, and you get to participate in the unfolding of that greatness.

The chapter on FAITH encouraged you to be a fearless advocate for your child. Fear can consume your energy, creativity, and spirit, disempowering you from taking the lead in your child's development. You must be relentless in confronting it and removing it from the fortress of your mind. Experience the joy of waking up every morning, full of energy and passion, knowing that you are equipped to play a key role in the life of your special child—a role that will enable your child to hone and deliver his innate gifts to the world. Dare to venture out of your circle of comfort to liberate your child's true human potential. Discipline, optimism, faith in your abilities, and an indomitable spirit will position you well as you progress on this unique path of self-discovery and empowerment.

You've learned that, as parents and guardians, it is our responsibility to help our kids reach and expand their capacity to live their best lives. We should be proactive in teaching our children the necessary life skills to become happy, independent adults who contribute to the world around them. Teach your children to run their race, competing only with themselves and measuring their success by seeing how far they've come.

While you wish to make life easier for your child, you've seen that it is significantly more critical to, proverbially, "teach the child to fish," maybe someday, they will even own the pond! Prepare them to do more for themselves. Prepare them to deal with challenges. Teach them to step out of their comfort zones to grow and go after their dreams and desires. They need to know that it's okay to be uncomfortable sometimes. Help your child face the world daily, armed with acquired tools. Some of our children will need support throughout their lives, but we should constantly strive and encourage them to be as independent as possible.

As you proceed to the GENTLE approach solution, you'll step up a gear while ensuring that your special child is fully on-board with you. Tenacity, strength of character, mental toughness and courage are key factors in developing persistence and finding success where others have yielded. And as you soldier on, you will find JOY to power your journey. Celebrate the small wins while you embrace and grasp every opportunity to teach. Flexibility is key—don't let your schedule be a shackle.

You've learned to let your child be a part of the process and take the lead whenever possible. You may not understand their actions, but you must recognise that only they know what they feel inside. Sometimes, you must step back and let your child lead you where they want to go.

You'll discover the need to be assertive but patient, to speak and listen, to support and be supported. As the LOVE game strategy comes alive, it becomes clear that this expedition is not a sprint but a marathon. Therefore, pausing for sustenance along the way is acceptable, provided you keep going and aim for continuous improvement.

You've learned the importance of embracing the individual your child is. They may be less outgoing, less articulate, or academically and socially less successful than you had expected. Maybe you had hoped for a quiet introvert, but you have a gregarious athlete. Perhaps you had wanted a teacher, but you got an artist instead. Life is like that; though we have free will and choice, we don't get to choose everything. Above all else, accept that your kid is different. Your child is living life on their terms and timeline, and the best you can do is appreciate their development, regardless of the pace. Every kid wants to be loved and accepted unconditionally by their parents. You've grieved the loss of the parenting experience and the child you had hoped for; now, you must be grateful for and enjoy your child.

Take time for enjoyment. The constant scramble between home, school, medical appointments and extra-curricular activities can be overwhelming. The pressures of balancing your many roles as parent, teacher, advocate, friend, and even therapist can be overwhelming, disconcerting, and exhausting. Remember to take moments for rest and renewal. Appreciate the simple moments with your child, knowing that you have been chosen as the custodian of this child. They might be differently abled, but this is part of what makes them who they are. Although their efforts and yours may often go unrecognized, the world is better because they're in it. Embrace your child and all the challenges and opportunities they have brought you with gratitude and love. Take heart and know that many out there fighting similar battles understand the depth of bravery and loyalty you have demonstrated.

Every one of us has the potential for extraordinary achievement, happiness and fulfillment. Our special children are no different. What lies behind pales in comparison when compared with what lies within. It takes small, consistent steps toward our dreams and goals. Lasting and profound change comes through the continued application of the approaches I shared with you and strategies you learn along the way. A meaningful life overflowing with wonders is built daily, and small wins lead to significant gains. Starting today, help your child learn more, live more and laugh more as you learn to love more. As you progress, you will arrive at a place of PEACE, knowing that you accomplished what was required of you.

Whether a parent, caregiver or educator of a special child, you will appreciate that finding balance and harmony despite the distinctive dynamics at play is not always easy. However, now that you have reached the end of this book, you can understand that this goal is achievable. And when you are successful, you'll realize that there is something magical and profound about being in a community that embraces individuals with special educational needs and disabilities.

I close with this quote by Zig Ziglar, "When you put faith, hope and love together, you can raise positive kids in a negative world." To that, I say - When you add gentleness, joy, and peace, you raise a balanced, confident child armed with the mindset, skills, and competencies to take his appropriate place in society. With hope providing a fitting foundation for the fruit of the spirit, your child—a fruit of the womb and fruit of your labor—will find his place in the world and all will be well.

A Note from the Author

Thank you so much for reading this book. I hope you enjoyed it and feel empowered to use everything you have learned. If you did, I would truly appreciate a useful review on Amazon. This way, other parents and guardians of children with special needs will benefit from reading this book, and will spread its message to others.

On that note, I love to hear from my readers! Feel free to reach out to me on social media sites or write to me via the contact page on Pocketlearner.net. Thank you so much!

Andrea Campbell

Other Books You'll Love

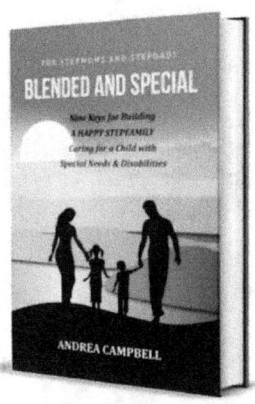

The 9-L model illustrated in "Blended and Special" explores the dynamics of stepfamilies caring for children with special needs and disabilities and presents the information in digestible nuggets ready for consumption by quintessential blended families juggling the demands of parenthood with caring for children with special needs.

https://amzn.to/3q8nO7F

(Amazon No. 1 Bestseller)

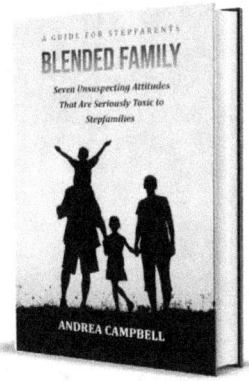

Blended Family – Seven Unsuspecting attitudes that are seriously toxic to stepfamilies outlines seven unempowering attitudes that seriously harm blended families, including those caring for children with special needs and disabilities. Available on Amazon.

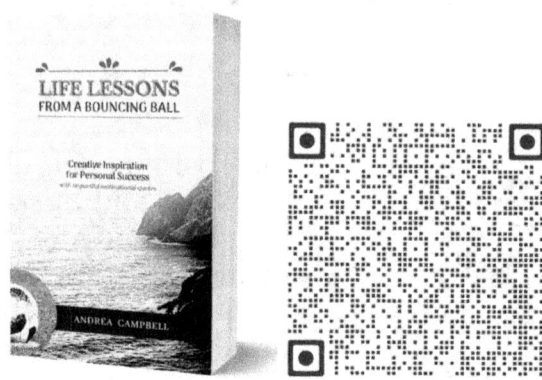

shorturl.at/cGTVW

Life Lessons from a Bouncing Ball – Creative inspiration and life lessons from a ball game.

About the Author

Andrea Campbell, MBA, MA, is a social entrepreneur, linguist, and inspirational writer. Since publishing her first book in 2010, Andrea has released several inspirational, business, cultural and personal development articles, including two Amazon No. 1 bestsellers.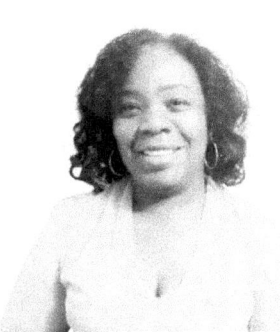

Over the years, she has focused on empowering vulnerable people through education and inspiration. As the mother of a child with special educational needs, she is particularly keen on working with families to enable their disabled children to aspire higher and achieve their potential. She is also the inventor of the Pocket Learner – a set of innovative educational resources for parents, caregivers, and educators of children with special educational needs.

A rather creative individual, Andrea has also published a range of inspirational coloring books, journals, and activity books to empower people everywhere.

Andrea resides with her family in London, UK, where she continues to have a positive impact through her writing, creative exploits, training programs, coaching, philanthropy, and inspirational speaking

Special Needs Glossary

Americans with Disabilities Act (ADA): a United States law passed in 1990 to protect people with disabilities from discrimination and to improve their access to services.

Assessment: a test or exam that collects information about a person's health or development. The results of an assessment can determine if a child is eligible for certain programs, services, or treatments.

Assistive technology: tools, devices, and aids designed to make everyday tasks easier for people with disabilities. Examples include bath seats, computers that read text aloud, weighted utensils, and pillbox reminders.

Beneficiary: a person named in a will, trust, or other agreement who will get financial benefits upon the death of the holder of the agreement.

Chronic: a lifelong condition, one that lasts for a long period of time, or one that happens again and again.

Cognitive: having to do with conscious mental activity, such as thinking, understanding, learning, and remembering.

Developmental disability: a condition that negatively affects a person's physical or mental abilities, including learning, language skills, and behavior. To be considered a developmental disability, the condition must start before age 22 and limit a person's ability to learn, live independently, use and understand language, earn a living, or be in charge of their own actions and care.

Early intervention services: a process that helps identify children with disabilities or developmental delays in the first years of life and provides them with the care they need to treat or prevent the disability or delay.

Functional life skills: learning that focuses on helping a person with a disability develop practical skills for living, such as cooking, shopping, doing laundry, and socializing.

Government benefits: help, in the form of money or services, that a person gets from the local, state, or federal governments. With health care, government benefits usually refer to Medicaid, Medicare, or a state-administered Children's Health Insurance Program (CHIP). Non-health care benefits include Supplemental Security Income (SSI) or Social Security Disability Insurance (SSDI).

Guardian: the person legally assigned to care for and be responsible for a child if the child's parents die before the child becomes an adult.

Home care: health care or assistance given to a person at home through a nurse or home health aide.

Home health aide: an individual who provides care in someone's home. Home health aides are trained in how to provide personal care, including bathing, dressing, feeding, and other daily routines.

Inclusion: the belief that people with disabilities should have the same access to services, activities, and opportunities as everyone else. For example, people with disabilities learn in regular (not separate) classes whenever possible and work in places designed to accommodate their disability.

Individualized education program (IEP): a written plan that outlines the educational goals and support needed for a student with disabilities. The IEP is agreed upon by the student's family, teachers, school administrators, and others.

Individualized Family Service Plan (IFSP): a personalized plan for young children with disabilities that outlines health and wellness goals and describes the steps that will be taken to reach those goals. The IFSP is developed by the child's family, doctors, and early childhood educators.

Individuals with Disabilities Education Act (IDEA): a 1977 federal U.S. law that helps guarantee no-cost educational services for children with disabilities.

Intellectual disability/intellectual disability disorder: a disability that limits a person's mental capacity (learning, problem-solving, reasoning) and adaptive behavior (language, social skills, daily activities). An intellectual disability starts before the age of 18.

Mainstreaming: when kids with disabilities spend time learning in regular classrooms and joining in activities alongside their peers without disabilities.

Medicaid: a state-run health care program that gets aid from the federal government to help people from low-income households or households with limited resources pay for medical costs. Medicaid is a form of health insurance. People need to meet the eligibility requirements to get Medicaid coverage in their state.

Motor development: changes in children's ability to control their movements. Gross motor development involves the large muscles in the legs, arms, and torso. Fine motor development involves smaller muscles like fingers, toes, lips, and tongue.

Occupational therapy: therapy that helps a person develop fine motor skills and learn daily living tasks such as writing, using eating utensils, and dressing.

Ombudsman: a person who investigates complaints and helps to settle them for a consumer.

Physical therapy: therapy that helps a child develop control of the large muscles involved in tasks like walking, sitting, standing, and lifting.

Placement: this can refer to the setting where a student with disabilities receives lessons or other educational services based on their individualized education program (IEP). It also can refer to "residential" placement, when a child lives in a place other than their natural home. This can be a group home, school, treatment facility, or other place.

Power of attorney: the legal right of a person (known as the "agent") to make decisions for an adult who cannot make them due to disability, illness, or distance. The adult who is handing over these powers must agree to this arrangement. Power of attorney rights can be short-term or long-term, and can be taken away at any time. The adult giving over this power still keeps their legal rights.

Regression: the loss of learned skills. For example, many kids regress over summer vacation or another time when they are away from instruction.

Respite care: a service that offers short-term care — from a few hours to a week or more — for a person with disabilities so the person's regular caregivers have time off.

Self-advocate: a person with disabilities who makes their own choices and decisions. Self-advocates speak up for themselves and others with disabilities.

Service provider: a person, organization, or business (for example, a hospital or childcare center) that provides assistive or medical services to a person with disabilities. The service provider can offer day programs, live-in aides, or residential services.

Social Security Disability Insurance (SSDI): a government benefit for adults with disabilities who have previously worked and paid into the government's Social

Security program. The benefit amount depends on how much and how long they paid into Social Security. This benefit can be used for any expenses, and there is no income limit for eligibility.

Special education services: education and therapy services provided to children with special needs at no cost to parents. The amount of services varies and depends on each child's needs and educational goals. Parents must ask for educational testing to see if their children are eligible for services.

Special needs trust: a financial trust, created by an estate or elder law attorney that allows someone with a disability to save money that does not count against his or her eligibility for government benefits like Supplemental Security Income (SSI) or Medicaid. Real estate, life insurance policies, and retirement savings all can be put into a special needs trust for someone with a disability, while still allowing the person to get government benefits.

Speech-language therapy: therapy that diagnoses and treats communication and speech problems.

Supplemental Security Income (SSI): a government benefit for anyone with disabilities who has little to no income, including children. SSI covers basic monthly expenses like room and board, clothing, and food. Eligibility is based on a person's income and assets.

Support services: services that allow students with disabilities to go to school. Support services include special transportation, medical services, and therapy.

Supported employment: a program that allows people with disabilities to work in a particular job while receiving support to help them complete the required tasks. Support can include specialized job training, job coaches, transportation, assistive technology, and other services that allow the person to get to and do the job.

Supported residential environment: a place where a person with a disability lives outside of their natural family home and gets help with activities of daily living (ADLs), managing treatments, and learning life skills. This place could be a group home, apartment, shared housing, or other housing.

Transition planning: a planned process for preparing a teen for early adulthood and beyond. This includes finding new doctors or other health care providers, taking a more active role in managing one's health care, and deciding where to live and work, if applicable.

Trust: a legal agreement in which a person or entity holds the right to manage property or assets for the benefit of someone else.

Trustee: the person responsible for managing a special needs trust for a person with disabilities after the death of that person's parents or legal guardian.

Vocational rehabilitation: a state-specific program that helps people with barriers to employment, including disabilities, get the training and support they need to get or keep jobs.

Waiver: for people with disabilities or chronic medical conditions - a request from their state to the federal government to remove restrictions on how Medicaid money is spent. Medicaid waiver programs help provide services to people who would otherwise be in an institution, nursing home, or hospital to receive long-term care in their communities.

Further Resources and Works Cited

1. 47 Stripey Socks. (2019, August 19). What I Love About Being the Parent of a Child with Special Needs. Firelyfriends.Com. Retrieved March 2, 2022, from https://www.fireflyfriends.com/ie/blog/what-i-love- about-being-the-parent-of-a-child-with-special-needs/

2. A P A. (2010, January). Disability and Social Economic Status. American Psychological Association. Retrieved March 2, 2022, from https://www.apa.org/pi/ses/resources/publications/disability

3. American Academy of Child and Adolescent Psychiatry. (2016, September). School Services for Children with Special Needs: Know Your Rights. AACAP. Retrieved March 2, 2022, from https://www.aacap.org/aacap/families_and_youth/facts_for_f amilies/fff-guide/Services-In-School-For-Children-With-Special-Needs-What-Parents-Need-To-Know-083.aspx

4. Ann, A. (2020, May 13). How to Nurture the Potential of Children with Special Needs. All In. Retrieved March 2, 2022, from https://allin.guide/blog/nurturing-children-with-special-needs/

5. Beurkens, N. D. (2017, July 7). The Importance of Optimism for Parents of Children with Special Needs. Dr. Beurken.Com. Retrieved March 2, 2022, from https://www.drbeurkens.com/the-importance-of-optimism-for-parents-of-children-with-special-needs/

6. Bikmal, H. B. (20202–06-01). The Value of Nurturing Your Special Needs Child's Hidden Talent. Autism Parenting. Retrieved March 2, 2022, from https://www.autismparentingmagazine.com/special-need-child-hidden-talent/

7. Children Educational Services. (n.d.). Five Tips for Helping Students with Special Needs. Retrieved March 2, 2022, from https://www.ces-schools.net/five-tips-for-helping-students-with-special-needs/

8. Cote, M. C. (2016, June 1). The Love I Have For My Child With Special Needs. Scary Mommy. Retrieved March 2, 2022, from https://www.scarymommy.com/love-child-special-needs/

9. Dear Special Needs Mom Ready to Give Up. (n.d.). Lemon Lime Adventures. Retrieved March 2, 2022, from https://lemonlimeadventures.com/dear-special-needs-mom-ready-to-give-up/

10. Driscoll, L. D. (2020, August 3). 9 Ways To Build Self-Confidence When Kids Have Learning Disabilities. Lorraine Driscoll. Retrieved March 2, 2022, from https://lorrainedriscoll.com/learning-disability-and-self-esteem/

11. Durand, M. D. (2011). Optimistic Parenting (1st ed., Vol. 1) [E-book]. Paul H Brooks.

12. Enable Group. (n.d.). What is a Learning Disability. Retrieved March 2, 2022, from https://www.enable.org.uk/get-support-information/what-is-a-learning-disability/

13. Enable Group. (n.d.-a). Developing Employment Skills. Retrieved March 2, 2022, from https://www.enable.org.uk/get-support-information/children-young-people/developing-employment-skills/

14. Family Monsters Project. (n.d.). Family Action Org. Retrieved March 2, 2022, from https://www.family-action.org.uk/family-monsters/support/supporting-children-with-a-learning-disabilities/

15. Fleming, N. F. (2020, March 27). New Strategies in Special Education as Kids Learn From Home. Edutopia. Retrieved March 2, 2022, from https://www.edutopia.org/article/new-strategies-special-education-kids-learn-home

16. FND. (n.d.). Florida's Resource for Helping Families of Children with Disabilities. Family Network on Disabilities. Retrieved March 2, 2022, from https://fndusa.org/

17. Hieneman, M.E.; Childs, K.; Sergay, J. (2008). Parenting with Positive Behavior Support (1st ed., Vol. 2) [E-book]. Paul H Brooks.

18. Kemp, Smith, Segal, G. K. M. S. J. S. (2020, November). Helping Children with Learning Disabilities. Help Guide. Retrieved March 2, 2022, from https://www.helpguide.org/articles/autism-learning-disabilities/helping-children-with-learning-disabilities.htm

19. Kemp, Smith, Segal, G. K. M. S. J. S. (2020, November). Learning Disabilities and Disorders. Help Guide. Retrieved March 2, 2022, from https://www.helpguide.org/articles/autism-learning-disabilities/learning-disabilities-and-disorders.htm

20. Kim-Kregel, P. (2011, February 2). Celebrating Children's Achievements Great and Small. Retrieved from https://www.greatschools.org/gk/articles/celebrating-achievements/

21. Linton, B. L. (2016, February 16). Learning Unconditional Love from Special Needs Children. The Good Men Project. Retrieved March 2, 2022, from https://goodmenproject.com/featured-content/learning-unconditional-love-from-special-needs-children-bbab/

22. Logsdon, A. L. (2020, August 30). Coping with Invisible Learning Disabilities. Very Well Family. Retrieved March 2, 2022, from https://www.verywellfamily.com/how-to-help-people-with-invisible-disabilities-cope-2162455

23. Loveless, B. L. (n.d.). 12 Strategies to Motivate Your Child to Learn. Education Corner. Retrieved March 2, 2022, from https://www.educationcorner.com/motivating-your-child-to-learn.html

24. Maxwel, N. M. (2021, July 23). Embracing your child with special needs just the way they are. Focus on the Family.

Retrieved March 2, 2022, from https://www.focusonthefamily.com/pro-life/embracing-your-child-with-special-needs-just-the-way-they-are/

25. McClafferty, J. M. (n.d.). 11 Classroom Management Strategies for Children with Special Needs. Stages Learning. Retrieved March 2, 2022, from https://blog.stageslearning.com/blog/11-classroom-management-strategies-for-children-with-special-needs

26. McGlensey, M. M. (2015, September 17). 23 Unique Lessons Parents of Children With Special Needs Have Learned. The Mighty. Retrieved March 2, 2022, from https://themighty.com/2015/09/23-unique-lessons-parents-of-children-with-special-needs-have-learned/

27. Medical causes of aggression in autism. The Autism Community in Action. https://tacanow.org/family-resources/medical-causes-of-aggression-in-autism/

28. Miller, J. M. (2019, August 28). The invisible part of special-needs parenting is what makes it so tough. Today's Parent. Retrieved March 2, 2022, from https://www.todaysparent.com/family/special-needs/the-invisible-part-of-special-needs-parenting-is-tough/

29. Mont, D. M. (2021). Combatting the Costs of Exclusion for Children with Disabilities and their Families (1st ed.) [E-book]. UNICEF.

30. National PTA. (n.d.). Special Education Toolkit Resources. Retrieved March 2, 2022, from https://www.pta.org/home/family-resources/Special-Education-Toolkit/Special-Education-Toolkit-Resources

31. Non-verbal learning disabilities. Learning Disabilities Association of America. (n.d.). Retrieved June 6, 2022, from https://ldaamerica.org/disabilities/non-verbal-learning-disabilities/

32. O'Shea, C. O. (2022, March). Individualized Education Programs. Kids Health. Retrieved March 2, 2022, from https://kidshealth.org/en/parents/iep.html

33. PACER. (n.d.). Top 10 Topics: Parents Concerns and Matching Resources. Pacer Center. Retrieved March 2, 2022, from https://www.pacer.org/parent/top10-parent-concerns.asp

34. PediaPlex. (n.d.). Encouraging Independence for Children with Special Needs. PediaPlex. Retrieved March 2, 2022, from https://www.pediaplex.net/blog/encouraging-independence-for-children-with-special-needs

35. Preuss, A. P. (n.d.). 3 Powerful Ways to Find Peace as a Special Needs Parent. Parents with Confidence. Retrieved March 2, 2022, from https://parentswithconfidence.com/the-3-keys-to-finding-peace-as-a-special-needs-parent/

36. Professional Organizations. Learning Disabilities Association of America. (n.d.). Retrieved March 2, 2022, from https://ldaamerica.org/resources/professional-organizations/

37. Raising Children Australia. (n.d.). Teaching skills to children with disability: practical strategies. Australian Parenting. Retrieved March 2, 2022, from https://raisingchildren.net.au/disability/school-play-work/learning-behaviour/teaching-skills-to-children-with-disability

38. Reframing Autism. (2018, October 18). The Gift of Unconditional Love. Retrieved March 2, 2022, from https://reframingautism.org.au/the-gift-of-unconditional-love/

39. Schaeffer, K. S. (2020, April 23). As schools shift to online learning amid pandemic, here's what we know about disabled students in the U.S. Pew Research Center. Retrieved March 2, 2022, from https://www.pewresearch.org/fact-tank/2020/04/23/as-schools-shift-to-online-learning-amid-pandemic-heres-what-we-know-about-disabled-students-in-the-u-s/

40. Sobsey, D. (2004). Marital stability and marital satisfaction in families of children with disabilities: Chicken or egg? Developmental Disabilities Bulletin, 32(1), 62-83. https://files.eric.ed.gov/fulltext/EJ848190.pdf

41. Support and Resources for Parents. Learning Disabilities Association of America. (n.d.). Retrieved March 2, 2022, from https://ldaamerica.org/audience/parents/

42. SSA. (n.d.). Social Security. Social Security Administration. Retrieved March 2, 2022, from https://www.ssa.gov/

43. Stumbo, E. S. (n.d.). How My Daughter With Down Syndrome Influenced My Writing. Ellenstumbo. Retrieved March 2, 2022, from https://www.ellenstumbo.com/blog/

44. The Importance of Affection in Children with Disabilities. (2019, September 18). You Are Mom. Retrieved March 2, 2022, from https://youaremom.com/children/what-should-you-know/tips-for-raising-your-child/children-disabilities/

45. The University of Washington. (2021, September 4). What is the difference between an IEP and a 504 Plan? DO IT. Retrieved February 20, 2022, from https://www.washington.edu/doit/what-difference-between-iep-and-504-plan#:~:text=The%20504%20Plan%20is%20a,access%20to%20the%20learning%20environment

46. Together for Children. (n.d.). Children With Disabilities. Retrieved March 2, 2022, from https://www.togetherforchildren.org.uk/parents-carers/children-disabilities

47. UK Government. (n.d.). Children with special educational needs. niDirect Government Services. Retrieved March 2, 2022, from https://www.nidirect.gov.uk/articles/children-special-educational-needs

48. UNICEF. (n.d.). 10 playful activities for children with disabilities. Retrieved March 2, 2022, from https://www.unicef.org/parenting/child-care/10-playful-educational-activities-children-disabilities

49. US Government. (2020, February 8). Benefits and Insurance for People with Disabilities. Retrieved March 2, 2022, from https://www.usa.gov/disability-benefits-insurance

50. Vanbuskirk, S. V. (2021, February 24). Why Its Important to Have High Self Esteem. Very Well Mind. Retrieved March 2,

2022, from https://www.verywellmind.com/why-it-s-important-to-have-high-self-esteem-5094127#toc-high-self-esteem

51. Washington University. (n.d.). Skip to main content DO-IT Disabilities, Opportunities, Internetworking, and Technology. DO IT. Retrieved February 20, 2022, from https://www.washington.edu/doit/

52. Words to Know (Special Health Care Needs Glossary) (for Parents) - Nemours KidsHealth. (n.d.). Kids Health. Retrieved July 18, 2022, from https://kidshealth.org/en/parents/special-needs-glossary.html

53. Wright, H. W. (2013). Complete Guide to Creating a Special Needs Life Plan: A Comprehensive Approach Integrating Life, Resource, Financial, and Legal Planning to Ensure a B (11th ed.). Jessica Kingsley Publishers.

54. Zensational Kids. (n.d.). The Power of Unconditional Love. Retrieved March 2, 2022, from https://zensationalkids.com/2013/03/01/the-power-of-unconditional-love/

55. Zubler, J. Z. (2021, April 10). Learning Disabilities & Differences: What Parents Need To Know. Healthy Children.Org. Retrieved March 2, 2022, from https://www.healthychildren.org/English/health-issues/conditions/learning-disabilities/Pages/Learning-Disabilities-What-Parents-Need-To-Know.aspx

www.ingramcontent.com/pod-product-compliance
Lightning Source LLC
Chambersburg PA
CBHW062113280426
43661CB00118B/1487/J